"For decades, Lacan's thought is proclaimed dead, outmoded by cognitive brain sciences or by 'non-binary' (trans, LGBT+) theories of sexuality – however, Lacan's theory simply refuses to die, haunting the entire humanities as an 'undead' creature. Is it possible to resume his writings which are proverbially ambiguous and unreadable? No, it's not possible – but in his *Jacques Lacan: the Basics*, Calum Neill does the impossible. Everyone can read and understand his book: it is like a top-quality trampoline, providing a firm basis on which each of us can do all the jumps and spins we want. So from now on there are no excuses permitted to those who continue to reject Lacan's theory as an unreadable mess – we should just simply respond them: 'But did you read Calum's book?' I have no doubts that thousands will."

Slavoj Žižek, *International Director of the Birkbeck Institute for the Humanities, Global Distinguished Professor of German at New York University, Professor of Philosophy at The European Graduate School and Senior Researcher at the Institute for Sociology and Philosophy at the University of Ljubljana.*

"This foundational text teaches us about Lacan in such a way as to also make clear that 'basic' need not simplify; this is an absorbing introduction that gives us something new while outlining what we need to know if we are to take next steps into Lacanian psychoanalysis."

Ian Parker, *Secretary, Manchester Psychoanalytic Matrix*

"Countless students and colleagues have asked for a guide to all things Lacan and beyond over the years. This is the book to recommend. While Lacan was wilfully difficult, he was not immune to moments of extraordinarily concision and clarity. Neill's introduction is a wonderfully effortless read. Lacan, in my mind, would have approved of this line thrown to open hands."

Jamieson Webster, *PhD Psychoanalyst and Clinical Psychologist*

"Calum Neill's introduction to the thought of Jacques Lacan is the only introduction that will ever be necessary. Written in the most welcoming and accessible manner, this book takes us on a journey into Lacan's theory with clear explanations and vibrant examples. Neill covers all the key points while providing enough depth that one can almost feel like an expert just after reading his work. This is *the* book to get before tackling Lacan or even instead of tackling Lacan."

Todd McGowan, *Professor of Film Studies, University of Vermont*

"An indispensable and much awaited guide for those wishing to find a way into the notoriously difficult oeuvre of Jacques Lacan. Dispelling the myths whilst staying true to the radical and challenging nature of his teaching, this book provides the tools needed to discover the relentlessly captivating and ever evolving world of Lacanian thought."

Isabel Millar, *Associate Researcher, Newcastle University*

JACQUES LACAN

Jacques Lacan: The Basics provides a clear and succinct introduction to the work of Jacques Lacan, one of the key thinkers of the 20th century. Lacan's ideas are applied in the study of the humanities, politics and psychology, as well as contemporary media and the arts, but their complexity makes them impenetrable to many. This book is unique in explaining the key concepts and context, from Lacan's understanding of psychoanalysis to drive and desire, in an accessible way without diluting them beyond meaning. Examples from popular culture are used throughout to emphasise the ideas being discussed, and a full glossary and list of resources for further reading are provided to encourage additional exploration.

This engaging and accessible text is essential reading for all those interested in Lacan and his work, including students of psychology, psychoanalysis, literature, politics, cultural studies, film studies and more.

Calum Neill is Associate Professor of Psychoanalysis and Cultural Theory at Edinburgh Napier University and the Director of Lacan in Scotland.

The Basics Series

The Basics is a highly successful series of accessible guidebooks which provide an overview of the fundamental principles of a subject area in a jargon-free and undaunting format.

Intended for students approaching a subject for the first time, the books both introduce the essentials of a subject and provide an ideal springboard for further study. With over 50 titles spanning subjects from artificial intelligence (AI) to women's studies, *The Basics* are an ideal starting point for students seeking to understand a subject area.

Each text comes with recommendations for further study and gradually introduces the complexities and nuances within a subject.

ANTHROPOLOGY
Peter Metcalf

ARCHAEOLOGY (SECOND EDITION)
Clive Gamble

ART HISTORY
Grant Pooke and Diana Newall

ARTIFICIAL INTELLIGENCE
Kevin Warwick

ATTACHMENT THEORY
Ruth O'Shaughnessy, Katherine Berry, Rudi Dallos and Karen Bateson

For a full list of titles in this series, please visit www.routledge.com/The-Basics/book-series/B

JACQUES LACAN

THE BASICS

Calum Neill

Routledge
Taylor & Francis Group
LONDON AND NEW YORK

Designed cover image: © Getty Images

First published 2023
by Routledge
4 Park Square, Milton Park, Abingdon, Oxon OX14 4RN

and by Routledge
605 Third Avenue, New York, NY 10158

Routledge is an imprint of the Taylor & Francis Group, an informa business

British Library Cataloguing-in-Publication Data
A catalogue record for this book is available from the British Library

Library of Congress Cataloging-in-Publication Data
Names: Neill, Calum, 1968– author.
Title: Jacques Lacan : the basics / Calum Neill.
Description: Abingdon, Oxon ; New York, NY : Routledge, 2023. |
Includes bibliographical references and index. |
Identifiers: LCCN 2022059255 (print) | LCCN 2022059256 (ebook) |
ISBN 9781138656222 (hardback) | ISBN 9781138656239 (paperback) |
ISBN 9781315622002 (ebook)
Subjects: LCSH: Lacan, Jacques, 1901–1981. | Psychoanalysts—
France—Biography. | Psychoanalysis—France—History—20th century. |
Philosophy—France—History—20th century.
Classification: LCC BF109.L28 N455 2023 (print) | LCC BF109.L28 (ebook) |
DDC 150.19/5092 [B]—dc23/eng/20230317
LC record available at https://lccn.loc.gov/2022059255
LC ebook record available at https://lccn.loc.gov/2022059256

ISBN: 978-1-138-65622-2 (hbk)
ISBN: 978-1-138-65623-9 (pbk)
ISBN: 978-1-315-62200-2 (ebk)

DOI: 10.4324/9781315622002

Typeset in Bembo Std
by codeMantra

For Claire and Atticus, with love

CONTENTS

ACKNOWLEDGMENTS

There is an obvious solitude in writing a book. You and a screen and other already existing books on hand. I had the good fortune to also have my cat, Stari, by my side for most of the writing of this book, and my other cat, Zuli, reminding me periodically that it was time to take a break. Beyond feline companions, however, there have been a number of people who, in their different ways, made the existence of this book possible.

First, and foremost, I want to thank Claire and Atticus. Your patience, support, encouragement and distractions made it all possible. It is simply a fact that without you, this book would never have been written.

I am also indebted to all the students who have questioned me and pushed me to try harder to explain Lacan throughout all the courses and classes I have taught. In particular, I am genuinely grateful to those students who didn't get it but who kept coming back and trying one more time. You know who you are.

There are three students I specifically want to thank and who deserve something far exceeding an acknowledgement. Anna, Antti and Claudia. You not only rose to the challenge of trying to understand Lacan but you took the risk of balancing your degrees on this wager. You excelled, but I know it cost you. You have my utmost respect. You are the kind of students who make the entire endeavour of teaching worthwhile. Thank you.

Thank you too to Amanda, my partner in crime at Lacan in Scotland, and former student. You sat through my classes, more times than anyone really ought to have to. And you kept coming back and pushing for better explanations and more clarity until you started to produce it yourself.

I am indebted to my good friend Derek Hook for the suggestion of *No Way Home* as an example of subjective destitution. And equally to my son, Atticus, for walking me through the nuances of the film, as well as puzzling over Descartes, Plato and Freud with me. Whatever education you do or don't gain at school, Atticus, you certainly provide me with one on our morning walks to get there.

Finally, this book was written in as much silence as I could achieve, but it was interspersed by entirely necessary bursts of Defcee and billy woods who soundtracked my runs in the rain and brought me back to the punctuated word. Maybe one day you will both read this book. Maybe not. But thank you anyway.

1

READING THIS BOOK

Jacques Lacan was a French psychoanalyst and teacher who lived and worked in Paris in the 20th century. He wrote very little but wielded an enormous influence both on the practice of psychoanalysis and on wider thinking around, amongst other things, our understandings of identity, ethics and social life. In addition to his rather small body of written work, most of it collected into two volumes (*Écrits*, meaning 'writings', and *Autre Écrits*, meaning 'other writings'), Lacan hosted regular lectures (referred to as seminars) which were transcribed and have, since 1975, begun to be published in French and subsequently in other languages, including English. Both the written work and the original oral presentations are dense and extremely challenging to read. The written work in particular is so formidable that it has led some to suggest that Lacan was simply not very good at writing. Others have suggested that he was wilfully obscure. The seminars are rather less dense than the works which were prepared for publication but are equally challenging to follow due to their lack of anything approaching obvious signposting. Lacan will often tell the audience at the beginning of the seminar what the seminar is about but then appears to wander somewhat freely from this point to the extent that it is rarely, if ever, clear where he is going or how each part of the unfolding lecture relates to what came before or what comes after. The fact, however, that so many remain enthralled by Lacan's work and that his influence over 20th and now 21st century thought remains significant suggests that, whatever the reason for the peculiar difficulty of his work, it is not that there is not something important being said in it.

DOI: 10.4324/9781315622002-1

There is a plausible reason for the difficulty presented in reading Lacan's work that is worth considering at the outset. The ideas that Lacan is trying to present are not themselves straightforward. Not only are they potentially provocative in their novelty, but they are also in danger of being misconstrued and subsumed within already accepted or known ideas. This is not a point particular to Lacan. It is, however, a point worth taking seriously, particularly in the context of this book. Whenever we encounter, for example, a new way of trying to conceive of our place in the world, we need to somehow fit that idea into or in relation to our already existing ideas of our relationship to the world. It would seem obvious that the more easily an idea fits with our old ideas, the less new it is. It may be a new idea to us but the fact that it can fit comfortably with the older ideas we have would suggest that this newer idea isn't really contesting those older ideas. In a sense, the older ideas have already paved the way for it. The idea itself tells us something new, but it conforms to the general understanding we have of ourselves, the world and the relationship between ourselves and the world. The more genuinely novel an idea is, the more challenging it is to accept. This is, in part at least, because it contests some of the older ideas we have relied upon. Such new ideas often require a new vocabulary to convey those aspects for which there previously were no concepts, no words. At other times, new ideas can be presented using new combinations of already existing words, or existing words which appear to be being used with a different sense.

The activity of fitting such new ideas into our already existing understanding, the activity of learning new things, new ways of seeing, can, therefore, be challenging or even uncomfortable. It is understandable then, that we might, without consciously thinking about it, tend towards the comfortable. That is to say, we might find ourselves forcing ideas to conform to the way of seeing the world to which we have already become accustomed. It is not that we don't want to learn new things, but the confusion and discomfort that comes with encountering brand-new ways of seeing can be unsettling. It suggests we may need to start to think everything from scratch all over again.

Added to this, when new ideas are presented in straightforward ways which accommodate easily to our conventional understanding, it is easy to mistake elements of these new ideas with seemingly similar ideas we have already encountered. Put in very simple terms, it is very easy to think we have understood something because we understand something which we think resembles it. This is rather how metaphors work. When we say, to give an apt example, that an idea is difficult to swallow, the metaphor works by conjuring an image. This image likely varies from person to person. It may be an image of a child taking medicine. The medicine is unpleasant to taste and thus causes a gag reflex. Or it may be an image of a snake attempting to devour whole another animal apparently bigger than itself. In both cases the images convey the sense of something being difficult to consume, to take into oneself. In the first example, this difficulty is due to the unpleasantness of the thing being consumed, even when we know it is in our own interest to consume it. In the second case, the difficulty is due to the mere size of the object. Both work to convey something of the challenge entailed in attempting to learn or accept new ideas. They may not be what we want to hear. They may simply be too enormous for us to take on.

While metaphors work rather well in this way to convey ideas more vividly, they also bring a risk. While a novel idea may be a bit like a spoonful of medicine, it is not actually a spoonful of medicine. Along with the points of comparison which help to convey the sense of challenge, the combination of the beneficial and the undesired, the metaphor also carries a bunch of potentially irrelevant or unhelpful images. The medicine example might give someone the idea that a new but unattractive idea can be made more attractive by following it with something more familiar and pleasant, such as a sweet. While this might work for actual medicine, it is less easy to see how this might work for ideas without the message starting to become confused. Moreover, the nature of metaphors is such that the precise image which is conjured is not really within our control. Are we supposed, in this instance, to imagine a child taking medicine, a snake eating an antelope or Cronos devouring his own offspring? The image to which we recourse affects the idea, which affects our understanding and we don't tend to purposively select the image in the moment. The image forces itself upon us depending on our prior experience and exposure.

Language can then be confusing as well as helpful, and this potential for confusion or misunderstanding is heightened in the case of novel ideas. It is, arguably, for this reason that Lacan (and he is not alone in this, particularly among French thinkers of the 20th century) writes in the way that he does. It is not simply that the ideas he is seeking to convey are novel and don't necessarily fit easily into our accustomed ways of seeing ourselves and our world. Lacan is very attuned to and concerned with the rush to comprehend that so often results in miscomprehension. He, therefore, presents his ideas in such a way as to make them less easy to grasp (and thus, arguably, less easy to misgrasp) on first (or second or third) reading. By presenting his ideas in such a way that you really have to consider what is being said, Lacan forces the reader to think and makes it less tempting to recourse to conventional ideas. He pushes you to think about how what is being said links to the other things being said. He asks you to think for yourself about what it might all mean, both in the sense of what the words say and in the sense of what the ramifications are of conceiving the self or the world in this or that way.

Lacan was a teacher. The aim of his work, then, is to encourage the reader to think for themselves. He doesn't tell you what to think. Sometimes it seems like he doesn't even tell you what he thinks. But he does push against other ways of thinking and does draw our attention to numerous concerns. He provides us with models, but even these models require interpretation. And this is rather the point. Lacan was a psychoanalyst. In this field everything must be interpreted. An important question in psychoanalysis is who does, or should do, the interpreting? A conventional assumption is that it is the job of the psychoanalyst to interpret. That is, after all, what we pay them for. Just as when you have a problem with your plumbing, you call a plumber and expect them to diagnose the problem and provide a solution, so when you visit a psychoanalyst, you might expect them to provide an interpretation of your experiences, a diagnosis of your problem and some sort of guidance or answer. This is a perspective that Lacan is keen to disrupt. From Lacan's perspective, the analyst is not the one who ought to provide an interpretation, never mind guidance. In fact, to put that more strongly, they ought to work hard not to provide an interpretation. Only you can interpret your experiences, dreams and desires. This shift of responsibility, for Lacan, occurs already at the level of the text. When you read, you are responsible for your reading, learning and interpretation of the text.

This book, then, is something of an impossibility. A failure before it is even written. The book sets out to provide some interpretations of Lacan. It sets out to try to put his still exceedingly challenging ideas into an accessible form. And it then, necessarily, encounters two problems from the outset. First, if Lacan wrote and presented his work in a purposively challenging way, to encourage his audience to think, then this book may appear to want to remove some of that challenge. Second, if the text of Lacan's work needs to be interpreted by the reader for themselves, then this book may appear to want to absolve you of that responsibility or ownership or worse, it may appear to want to impose another interpretation which forever colours your own. These failings are, perhaps, unavoidable in a text like this. As an introduction to Lacan, it has to put forward ways of understanding him and has to reframe and simplify some of his ideas. The book proclaims to present the basics, when arguably there is nothing basic about Lacan and the basis of his ideas requires some really heavy work of digging.

In a sense, then, there are two options. You might want to stop reading here and simply pick up one of Lacan's own books and start with that. The problem is that this option has defeated some worthy adversaries. It is not an easy option, although it is not an impossible option. But the choice is yours. The second option, I suggest, is that you use this book but you remind yourself, while reading and once you have read it, that it simplifies, misrepresents and that it arises through a particular reading of Lacan, informed upon by a particular readerly context, a context which will not be yours.

Lacan used to refer, jokingly (which is not to say without seriousness), to his writings as *poubellication*. This is a made-up word, a play on the French words *poubelle*, meaning 'bin,' and *publication* (it's the same in French). Lacan appears to be making a connection between publishing his ideas and discarding them. In a more obvious way, I would like to retrieve this notion of *poubellication* and suggest that once you have read this book, you discard it. You might want to pass it on to someone else rather than throw it in the bin. The choice is yours. Either way, I suggest you make what use you can of the explanations offered, but, once you have got the gist, you dispense with the book and the ideas within it and begin the real journey of reading Lacan yourself.

CHAPTER SUMMARY

In this chapter, we have explored some suggestions for how to read or treat the book. The key ideas covered are:

- Encountering new ideas can be challenging.
- All reading is an act of interpretation.
- You should be ready to discard the interpretations offered in this book and formulate your own.

2

WHO WAS JACQUES LACAN?

Given that Lacan was a psychoanalyst, it might be tempting to begin by exploring his childhood, his family, looking for some kind of seed of who he became in those formative days and relations, but I'm inclined to skip all that David Copperfield kind of crap. Tempting as it might be to draw threads back into versions of Lacan's personal history, it would only be conjecture. It is, however, perhaps helpful to have a little bit of context, some orientation.

Lacan was born in Paris in 1901 and lived, studied and worked there until his death in 1981. He trained initially as a medical doctor (and later became Pablo Picasso's personal physician) before specialising in the still rather new discipline of psychiatry. As a branch of medicine, psychiatry follows a medical framework. Just as in general medicine, conditions are identified and, where possible, treatments are advanced. The patient in this framework is rather like an object, something which needs correcting or fixing in order to function more normally. And just as medicine has evolved over centuries, with significant leaps forward occurring with the advent of modern science and technology, so too our understanding of the mind and human behaviour has changed over time. Psychiatry as an established medical discipline was less than a century old when Lacan embarked upon his studies, but people had been exploring and explaining madness, deviance and difference for millennia. As a new discipline, and particularly as a new discipline seeking to explain and treat phenomena which were rather difficult to pin down, there was (and still is) no one way of doing psychiatry, no one set of understandings. There was, however, a general perspective which sought to

DOI: 10.4324/9781315622002-2

position the exploration of madness and mental abnormality within the broader discipline of medicine and, thus, as an applied science.

Sigmund Freud, like Lacan, had originally studied medicine and had then been drawn, through an interest in neurology, to psychiatry. Through his explorations and particularly through his work with patients, Freud began to develop a practice which departed in significant ways from psychiatry. While there is no space here to engage in a full and detailed comparison of psychiatry and psychoanalysis, it is worth noting two key and interrelated points of distinction. Psychiatry and psychoanalysis, while ostensibly focused on the same area of study – the mind, human behaviour, madness, deviance, etc. – operate with quite different sets of assumptions. That is to say, the understanding of what the mind is and how it works is based on different theories. This then connects to a second distinction: the two disciplines, in practice, rely on quite different ways of positioning the person who is being treated and even, then, the very notion of what would count as and what would be the aim of 'treatment.' A medical model most obviously aims to provide a cure or, at the very least, some system of management for an ailment. Such an approach relies on a notion of what is healthy or normal. The job of the psychiatrist then, as an external expert, is to identify the problem and provide a cure, treatment or, at least, containment. Frustrated with what he saw as the limitations of this approach, Freud sought to approach the mind from a different perspective. Importantly, Freud did not set out with a clear set of assumptions so much as with a powerful inquisitiveness. His explorations and, crucially, his explorations with his patients led him to a number of novel ideas and the establishment of a new discipline he called psychoanalysis.

Possibly the most well-known novelty of Freud's approach and one of the things that distinguishes it from psychiatry is the invention of the unconscious. I say 'invention' rather than 'discovery' because what Freud was doing was concocting an explanatory framework rather than uncovering an already existing entity. We can already see here how this begins to distinguish his approach from a more medical perspective. The other well-known and obvious, and rather related, novelty of Freud's approach was the emphasis he placed on the patient's speech. Psychoanalysis became known as the talking cure, a term actually coined by one of Freud's early patients, which also then serves to emphasise the place or role of the patient in the treatment. Psychoanalysts, reflecting this distinction, also tend not to use the term 'patient.' Instead, they refer to the person working with the psychoanalyst as an analysand.

Freud's first forays into psychoanalysis were towards the end of the 19th century. By the 1920s, his ideas had become fairly well-known and talked about.

As a pioneer, it is important to keep in mind that Freud's ideas were constantly evolving. If you read Freud's many essays and books, what jumps out most readily is his own questioning of his own ideas. He doesn't settle. And it wasn't only Freud who was questioning his ideas. He soon attracted an active following of others adopting this psychoanalytic approach and adopting too the need to explore further these new ideas, questioning and developing, adapting and overturning theories and practices.

By the time Lacan was undertaking his psychiatric training, Freud's ideas had arrived in France and specifically French approaches to psychoanalysis were beginning to emerge.

Lacan had already developed an interest in Freud's work before he completed his training, and there is a clear influence of psychoanalytic thinking on his thesis, which was submitted and published in 1932. While his thesis is a work of psychiatry, which does engage with and extend psychoanalytic ideas, it is not yet really a work of psychoanalysis. When Lacan sent his completed thesis to Freud, Freud gave no sign of having read it.

A peculiarity of psychoanalysis is that it is considered essential to undergo psychoanalysis yourself before you can become a psychoanalyst. The same year Lacan submitted his psychiatric thesis, just as he was writing up his final draft, he also entered into analysis with the Polish analyst Rudolph Lowenstein. From this point on, we can understand Lacan as having made the shift from psychiatry to psychoanalysis. Like many psychoanalysts or psychoanalytic thinkers, and like Freud before him, Lacan was not content to simply absorb and practise a discipline as was. From the outset, he was engaging with and developing the ideas and very much beginning to establish his own perspective and style. Although he wrote and published before this, what is often marked as Lacan's 'coming out,' or significant moment, took place in Marienbad in August 1936 when he presented his ideas on what came to be known as 'the mirror stage' to the Congress of the International Psychoanalytic Association

(IPA). His presentation was cut short by Ernest Jones, possibly simply because he, Lacan, ran over his allotted time, although the incident is often presented as exemplifying Lacan's already emerging outsider status in relationship to the mainstream movements of psychoanalysis.

It is worth emphasising the plural here: movements. Although Freud is still alive at this point and the ideas of psychoanalysis are still really rather new, the field has already begun to split into different schools or different perspectives. Jung, probably the most famous of Freud's one-time followers, had stepped away from many of Freud's teachings as early as 1912. Many other psychoanalysts developed their own theories from Freud's theories, and the field has continued to split, often acrimoniously, ever since, often with divergent factions each claiming to be the true followers of Freud. On the one hand, we can see Lacan's emergence as an original thinker within the psychoanalytic field as simply one of many, but there is also the sense in which his split was particular. Despite their many differences and innovations, many of the different schools would still associate with and share membership of wider organisations like the IPA.

The ideas Lacan presented about his notion of a mirror stage in 1936 were never published in their original form. Lacan claimed to have lost the paper. The theory of the mirror stage is, however, developed over a number of years, appearing in what is understood to be close to the form he presented in 1936 in an Encyclopaedia entry that Lacan published in 1936. He further worked the ideas and in 1949 eventually published the now well-known version as 'La stade du miroir comme formateur de la function du Je telle qu'elle nous est révéléle dans l'expérience psychanalytique' ('The Mirror Stage as Formative of the Function of the I as Revealed in Psychoanalytic Experience'). This short essay – it is only seven and a half pages long – contains a wealth of novel ideas and truly sets Lacan apart from his contemporaries. Lacan, like Freud before him, never settled. He constantly reviewed, questioned and developed his own ideas. It is difficult, therefore, to pin some aspects of his theory down and impossible to talk of a singular, definitive Lacanian theory. The 'Mirror Stage' essay does, however, contain the seeds or foreshadowing, of many, although, of course, not all, of the ideas Lacan would go on to develop.

Four years after the publication of the 'Mirror Stage' article and 17 years after his presentation at Marienbad, Lacan and many of his followers broke away from their governing institution, the *Parisian Society of Psychoanalysis* (SPP) and formed the *French Society of Psychoanalysis* (SFP). While this can all sound a little like a scene from *Monty Python's The Life of Brian,* the differences behind the split are not trivial. Lacan, you will recall, has moved progressively away from the medical model upheld by psychiatry, and the split of 1953 was largely in response to the SPP's perceived turn back towards this medical model. Psychoanalysis is a practice, but it is a practice very much predicated on a theory and Lacan took this theory and the need to interrogate it, develop it and reshape it, very seriously.

Also in 1953, Lacan began to host a weekly seminar in Paris. Not only did this platform serve to further establish Lacan as a prominent figure, an intellectual leader and a teacher, but it also served to provide the clearest documentation of his developing ideas. His seminars ran more or less continuously for 27 years and have since been published or made unofficially available. Eleven years into his seminar, 11 years after the establishment of the SFP, Lacan once again found himself on the outside. The SFP was keen to secure International Psychoanalytic Association (IPA) recognition as a training institute. This kind of recognition was, within the psychoanalytic world, a significant marker of status. The IPA agreed to welcome the SFP as a member organisation on one condition, that they expel Lacan from their number.

Lacan's crime had been to question, and practically contravene, one of the key orthodoxies of psychoanalytic practice. Despite all the theoretical differences, developments and disputes between the various psychoanalytic factions, they all maintained a peculiar allegiance to what is known as the 'psychoanalytic hour.' When Freud had first established the practice of psychoanalysis, he had adopted the pattern of meeting with his clients for an hour at a time. This kind of makes sense from a straightforward organisational perspective. You want to organise your day and your clients. Like a dentist or an estate agent, it makes life easier if the people seeing you have clear appointments and for one person to have a clear start time, the person before would obviously need to have a clear finish time. You also require a little bit of a buffer zone between the two clients: time for one to leave and the other to arrive (and allegedly, time for Mrs Freud to water the plants in Freud's study). Freud, therefore, established the psychoanalytic hour, a conventional 50 minute session. While this approach might make perfect sense for a dentist or an estate agent, it brings with it a significant problem for psychoanalysis.

The practice of psychoanalysis involves lying on a couch and speaking freely, or free associating. The idea is that you, the analysand, unshackle your thoughts from the usual self-censorship that you would normally apply. This might sound easy enough, but in practice, it is really rather hard to do. Not only are we accustomed to quite consciously hold back some of what we might say, out of propriety, convention or embarrassment, but there is also, in the context of psychoanalysis, the unconscious to consider.

Arguably, the whole of Freud's theory relies on the idea of the unconscious. That is, the idea that there is a part of us, a force or structure within us, that is not within our control. Freud argued that some ideas were too unpleasant, painful, threatening or confusing for the conscious mind to handle. These ideas would then be repressed. How exactly we conceive of the unconscious is a complex issue to which we will return. Using spatial or physical metaphors to discuss the unconscious is rather misleading. But it is also helpful. So, keeping in mind that the unconscious is not a place in your head, just as the mind is not the brain, let us imagine it as a storeroom of unmanageable ideas. Repression is the activity of consigning these difficult thoughts to this repository. The difficult thoughts, however, don't want to stay in the repository, so they will emerge in various moments, through slips of the tongue (when you say what you really mean rather than what you meant to say) and through dreams (where they appear as nonsense). There is then something like an ongoing internal struggle, with the unconscious working to keep the difficult thoughts repressed and the difficult thoughts working to find expression. Part of the work of psychoanalysis, through the mechanism of free association, is to allow the difficult thoughts to emerge.

Lacan realised that, if you maintain a strict and predictable duration for the psychoanalytic session, you are effectively providing the unconscious with a huge advantage. If you know that you have to talk for 50 minutes and there is something you really don't want to talk about, you can imagine how easy it would be to protract your narrative, or wander off topic, until your time is up. If you kind of do want to talk about something but are also rather nervous about talking about it, you might then talk around it for forty-nine and a half minutes and then briefly mention it just at the point when you know the session is about to end. Not only is this quite likely to happen on a very conscious level, Lacan was aware that it is even more likely to happen on an unconscious level. The unconscious, as it works to maintain repression, can also utilise the clock, timing the release for just the point at which nothing more can be explored or simply timing how long the free association needs to be endured without saying anything of any import. Lacan, therefore, began to introduce, and to advocate amongst his followers, what he called the 'short session.' The name is a little misleading as Lacan was not necessarily suggesting that the sessions needed to be shorter. What he was suggesting was that the analysand needed to be cut short (rather as he had been in Marienbad). His idea was that, if the analysand, and therefore the analysand's unconscious, didn't know how long the session was going to last, they could no longer play the session to their advantage (which, of course, within the aims of psychoanalysis, isn't really to their advantage at all). The psychoanalyst could sit and let the analysand talk and talk until they exhausted themselves and started to allow the unconscious to speak. Or, when the analysand was simply intent on talking conventionally about themselves (what Lacan calls 'ego speech'), the analyst could cut them off, effectively saying, I am not interested in this superficial rambling. Or, thirdly, the analyst could, by rejecting the 50 minute convention, carefully utilise the ending of the session to draw the analysand's attention to something. An important aspect of psychoanalysis is that the work of analysis doesn't only happen in the session with the analyst. You inevitably come away from the session thinking about what you have said, what your analyst has and hasn't said, the particular point at which they coughed and the lack of any comment after you divulged what you thought was your most significant secret. Aspects of the dream you recounted return, more vividly or more connectedly than before, in the hours or days after the session. Suddenly, the nonsense you could make no sense of will start to make some sense, or the sense you thought you had made will start to dissolve into nonsense, to be picked up anew at your next session. By rejecting the hourly convention, Lacan made the timing of the session an active part of the analysis itself, part of the directing of the treatment. He allowed himself to punctuate the analysis.

This innovation is perhaps the most concrete and identifiable of Lacan's deviations from the International Psychoanalytic Association orthodoxy, but it was not the only one. Moreover, Lacan himself was part of the problem. A charismatic leader, as well as a fierce innovator, Lacan commanded considerable loyalty from his followers, many of whom had undertaken analysis with him. This loyalty appears to have been based on a mixture of the personal and the intellectual. That is to say, while some of Lacan's followers appeared to be following him, others appeared to be following his ideas and, most likely, most were drawn by a mixture of the two. More than simply some gossip concerning Lacan's style or personality, this distinction is rather important here. There is no doubt that Lacan was a flamboyant figure. He was unusually intelligent and not a little arrogant. He appears to have been very concerned about his own position within the psychoanalytic community and within the French intellectual world beyond psychoanalysis. At the same time, his ideas and constructive critiques of Freudian theory and practice were rigorously thought through and grounded in a profound ethical thinking. Whatever part Lacan's attitude, demeanour and behaviour played in affecting the psychoanalytic establishment's view of him, the impact of his ideas cannot be diminished.

After a protracted process of review and deliberation, in 1963 the IPA agreed to recognise the SFP but on the condition that Lacan and a number of others were excluded.

As already noted, Lacan had begun to deliver a weekly seminar in 1953. These took place at Sainte-Anne Hospital, a psychiatric hospital and centre of teaching in Paris. When Lacan was expelled from the SFP in 1963, he was forced to cut short his seminar and find a new location. He turned to the renowned Marxist philosopher Louis Althusser who was able to arrange for him to continue his seminars at the *École Normale Superieure*, the home of such well-known thinkers as Sartre, Derrida, Foucault and Bourdieu. This shift in location might also be understood as a shift in Lacan's reception. His ideas and his influence went from being focused on and taken up by psychoanalytic practitioners to gaining a wider audience among the intellectuals of Paris. After the Paris uprisings of 1968, Lacan had to move his seminar again, this time to the University of

Paris. While his writing and teaching never lost their focus on the practice of psychoanalysis, it is clear from his reception by the intellectual and academic, rather than psychoanalytic, establishment that what he had to impart reached far beyond the interests of clinical practitioners.

This breadth of reach was always there in Lacan's influences and the many, often obtuse, references he made in his articles and seminars. Freud's work had always contained the imprint of the influence of philosophy, even if it wasn't always direct. Much of Freud's theoretical direction can be seen as following in the wake of the ideas of the 19th-century German philosopher Arnold Schopenhauer. Schopenhauer broadly anticipated many of the ideas which we have come to understand as Freudian, such as the role of repression, the structure of the psyche and even that most Freudian of concepts, the Freudian slip (or parapraxis, to give it its proper name). Freud famously denied having read Schopenhauer until later in his life, after he had developed the theories that appear to contain echoes of Schopenhauer's thought. It may be, however, that the influence of Schopenhauer came through other writers with whom we know Freud to have been familiar, such as Friedrich Nietzsche.

Lacan's knowledge of philosophy is much more overt, and the influence is in many ways much clearer. As a young man he studied Spinoza. Later, he attended lectures by Alexandre Kojève, who is credited with introducing Hegel to a whole generation of French intellectuals and who had himself floated the idea of a synthesis of Freudian and Hegelian ideas. Lacan evidently read widely and deeply and even employed a private philosophy tutor. Arguably, it is this engagement with philosophy that allowed Lacan to develop in a direction quite distinct from his medical-psychiatric beginnings. Lacan's works are always focused on psychoanalysis, and they often entail direct engagements with Freud's texts. But they are also often focused on philosophy and entail direct engagement with the works of Descartes, Plato, Hegel, Wittgenstein, etc. Moreover, the circles Lacan was moving in, the vibrant intellectual climate of Paris, included many philosophers – such as Sartre, Deleuze and Derrida – who engaged with Lacan's work and with whose work Lacan in turn engaged.

A core question, which arguably dominated early 20th-century French philosophical circles, was the question of subjectivity; i.e., what does it mean to be a person? It is not hard to see how this question bridges both philosophy and psychoanalysis. Much of Lacan's significance lies in his efforts to answer – or theorise – this matter, to produce a new, coherent theory of the subject.

CHAPTER SUMMARY

In this chapter, we have briefly explored aspects of Lacan's background and how his work fits into the development of the discipline of psychoanalysis. The key ideas covered in the chapter are:

- Psychoanalysis, unlike psychiatry, does not follow a medical model.
- Key among the novelties of psychoanalysis are the idea of the unconscious and the emphasis placed on speech.
- Lacan's ideas, which were continuously developing, stand apart from other forms of psychoanalysis.
- A significant distinction between Lacan's version of psychoanalysis and other versions was his discarding of conventional session lengths. This move allowed him to make the timing of the session part of the analysis itself. It also got him kicked out of the main psychoanalytic organisation, the International Psychoanalytic Association.
- Lacan's ideas extend beyond psychoanalysis, drawing in influences from philosophy and finding an audience in philosophical as well as psychoanalytic circles.
- The question of subjectivity is one which bridges both psychoanalysis and philosophy and Lacan's theory of subjectivity is one of his most significant contributions to world thought.

3

SOME PHILOSOPHICAL CONTEXT

Let's begin with Descartes. European philosophy clearly doesn't start with Descartes, but Descartes charged himself with the task of starting it again, supposedly from scratch. Descartes was born at the end of the 16th century and lived in France and Holland until his death in 1650. This was a tumultuous time in European intellectual life. For some six centuries, Europe had lived under a feudal system and been dominated by the Roman Catholic church. This combination of social and religious structures meant that European society was strictly hierarchical. If you were a peasant, you would have been illiterate, educated only in the practice of the crafts with which you were expected to work and destined to a rather brief life of poverty. The concept of social mobility simply didn't exist. If you were born a peasant, you would live as a peasant and die a peasant. You may have found yourself conscripted to fight in an army but that would not have been a choice, or not your choice. If you were born into a merchant family, you would have enjoyed a more affluent life, but not really much more choice or freedom. Higher up the social hierarchy, people would have more power, but the notion that you were born into your place in society was fundamental. A similar hierarchy structured the religion of the time, Roman Catholicism. At the top of the hierarchy was God, beneath God, the Pope, the cardinals, bishops, priests and below the priests, the people. As literacy was the preserve of the wealthy and the church, the word of God (the Bible), like so much else, was only available to those at the top, who would pass it down to – or determine it for – those below.

The philosophy of Europe in this period was similarly controlled by the church. As the clergy and aristocracy would have been the

DOI: 10.4324/9781315622002-3

only ones with access to literacy and books, the production of and interpretation of ideas almost exclusively emerged from the Christian tradition. The two most significant thinkers of this period were St Augustine and St Thomas Aquinas. Augustine was born into a wealthy family in North Africa and became a teacher of rhetoric, or argumentation. Although his mother was a Christian, it was only later that he himself turned to Christianity, was baptised, then ordained and eventually became the Bishop of Hippo (in what is now Algeria). Augustine wrote a lot, and through his writing, he strongly influenced the theology of Europe for centuries after his own death. Although Augustine apparently never mastered Greek himself, his ideas were very influenced by Plato. At the risk of being reductionist, we might say that he took the basics of Platonic philosophy and blended them with Christianity, giving Christianity a more solid or thought-through foundation in the process. Looked at from a different angle, we might also say that he allowed Plato's ideas to persist in a Christian dominated society.

Augustine also, curiously, bequeathed to us what is arguably the world's first autobiography in the form of his *Confessions*. The *Confessions* are notable in that they present the life of an individual with a sense of purpose and with an individual trajectory. This may seem a rather obvious idea to us, in the 21st century, when every bookshop is choked with celebratory autobiographies and the idea of the individual life as being a coherent and discrete journey is widely accepted. In the 4th century, however, this idea was far from obvious. Most people's lives weren't really much of a journey, and, moreover, we have little reason to believe that it would have been thought about that way. If you have no choice, it is difficult to see in what sense your life could be conceived as a meaningful journey. It is also worth noting, in the context of thinking about psychoanalysis, that the life Augustine tells in his *Confessions* is just that, a telling. It is a story. This is not to suggest that it is not true, but true or not, a story requires selection and structuring and putting into words. This is rather like what happens in the psychoanalytic clinic.

Although often thought together, Thomas Aquinas lived around 900 years after Augustine. Like Augustine, he was strongly influenced by Greek thought. Where Augustine's ideas can be thought of as a Christianising of Platonism, Aquinas's favoured source was Plato's student, Aristotle. He wrote explicitly on Aristotle, producing commentaries and interpretations of key Aristotelian ideas but also producing original work which bears the influence of Aristotle. A key example here might be Aquinas's ideas about the soul and the body. Following Aristotle, Aquinas argues that the soul and the body are distinct and that it is only in their combination that we can describe someone as human. A dead body is, therefore, strictly speaking, ex-human, rather than human, as the soul would have departed. Aristotle had made the distinction between matter and form – the stuff something is made of and the shape it is made into. Plasticine, we might think of as the matter. The form is all the various things you can make out of the plasticine. A human body (or potentially human body) only becomes a human body when the material substance is combined with a soul. The soul, for Aquinas, is a substantial form but not a substance itself. It is the thing that transforms the material of the body into a specific human entity. It is the soul then that sets the human apart. Again, following Aristotle, Aquinas argues that the human is uniquely positioned as a rational being. It is the soul that encapsulates this rational dimension.

We can see here that the influence of Aristotle, through Aquinas, affects not only what we might think of as obviously religious matters but spills over into our understanding of or explanation of the world itself.

Aristotle had been a profound polymath. He wrote not only on ethics and politics but also on language, physics and the natural world. He categorised plants and animals, and many of the categories he established remain in use today. His ideas on the elements and physical properties remained in place throughout the medieval period. Aristotle had proposed that the world is composed of five basic elements: fire, water, earth, air and aether. Anything solid is largely composed of earth. Anything liquid is largely composed of water. And so on. Aristotle further proposed an explanation for gravity. He argued that each element's tendency is towards its own natural resting place among its own type. Fire, then, moves upwards towards the sun, as is easily observed if we strike a match. Water and earth will move downwards. Spill a glass of water, and it will run off the table and fall to the floor. If possible, it will run to a drain, to the sewerage system and eventually to the sea. An apple, or any solid object, will simply fall to the ground and will continue falling, or rolling, as low as it can. It is kind of easy to see the attractiveness of this theory of gravity. It has a certain sense to it. It has, however, been supplanted by Isaac Newton's explanation, which better explains the uniformity of gravity and the fact, for example, that heavier and lighter objects fall at the same rate.

Newton's work appeared shortly after Descartes died but can be understood as part of a trajectory of change in European thought which had been progressing rapidly for a couple of hundred years.

In 1440, Johannes Gutenberg had invented the moveable printing press which began a major revolution in the communication of ideas. Until this point, all writing had been literally that, writing. Books were reproduced through the laborious work of hand copying. As this work was undertaken by monks, it is easy to see the stranglehold the church maintained on what could and could not be reproduced. Added to which, most people couldn't read and, as all the books had to be handwritten, there weren't that many books to read.

The domination of the Roman Catholic Church was brought significantly into question in 1517 when Martin Luther produced his 95 Theses, 95 points with which he took issue concerning the practices and beliefs of the Catholic Church. Remember that the church was a strict hierarchy, with what we might understand as a series of gatekeepers between the people and God. The Pope could communicate directly with God. The Pope would then communicate with the cardinals, who would communicate with the bishops, who would communicate with the priests, who would eventually sermonise to the people. Amongst other things, Luther objected to this hierarchy, arguing that each man was his own pope. That is to say, each of us has direct access to God. This is not a simple disagreement about the nature of God. It rocked the very foundations of the church and gave rise to a new form of Christianity called Protestantism.

The emergence of this new way of thinking about our relation to God in conjunction with Guttenberg's printing press meant the widespread dissemination of an alternative understanding of people's place in the world. Transposing the argument against the church hierarchy and in favour of individual responsibility to the state, we can see the seeds of modern democracy begin to sprout. Significant parts of Europe began to separate from the authority of the church, giving rise to the Thirty Year War.

Not only was people's relation to God and their place in the world beginning to be brought into question but the nature of the world itself and its place in the universe was being rethought. In 1543, Nicolaus Copernicus published his treatise on heliocentrism. Heliocentrism is the idea that the sun is at the centre of things. Up until this point, European thought had been strictly geocentrist, that is, believing that the earth was the centre of everything. Again, the dominance of the church is important here. The Bible presents the idea that God created man in his own image, thus suggesting that man is the most important of His creations. The Earth, being man's home, is obviously, then, the most important place in the universe. It makes sense, then, that physically everything revolves around the Earth, just as conceptually everything revolves around man. By questioning the former, Copernicus implicitly questions the latter. It took some 70 years for the full impact of Copernicus's ideas to hit the church, when his ideas were developed and defended by Galileo Galilei.

By the time of Descartes, these developments in theology, philosophy, the natural sciences and politics had begun to be accepted and it was widely understood to be a time of liberation of thinking, a period, as it came to be known, of enlightenment. It was the beginning of what we understand as modern science, the beginning in many ways of what we understand as the modern world. It was in this context that Descartes came to the conclusion that he needed to begin philosophy again.

So much was changing in the way that the world was understood that Descartes figured that he would be wise to question everything. If, he reckoned, so much of what he had been taught as true had been shown to be false, then there was literally nothing that he could take for granted. It seemed quite likely that even the things which had not been shown to be false might well turn out to be so. He set about, then, constructing a new philosophy, one which did not rely on the teachings of those who had come before.

His new philosophy, or the basis of it, is captured in his *Meditations on First Philosophy*. The book is written as a series of six meditations or thought experiments and is presented rather like a diary. On the first day, he sets out the issue, the fact that nothing he has hitherto learned can be trusted. He extends this doubt, beyond what he has learned, to his own immediate experience. When he is dreaming, he says, he experiences a world which he takes, in the dream, to be reality. How then can he ever be sure that he is not in a dream?

Any evidence he finds to establish the reality of the world around him and his experience of it might just be part of the dream as well. So, he sets out to doubt everything until he can find something of which he can be certain. He doubts his learning, his senses, the world around him and the reality of other people. Everything. But he then realises that no matter how much he doubts, one thing appears to remain true, that he is engaged in this process of doubting. This appears to suggest that, despite all the doubt, he must have some reality, insofar as he is having all these doubts.

On the second day, he tests this idea with the suggestion that it is perhaps not he himself who is having these thoughts of doubt, that perhaps some evil demon is putting these thoughts into him. This is essentially the basis of the Wachowskis's film *The Matrix*. In the film, Neo discovers that his entire existence is fake and that he is really in a comatose state in a pod, plugged into a malevolent AI network which generates what he (and, by extension, we) take to be reality. Even in this level of reality, though, Descartes concludes that he must exist, even if he only exists as the receptacle of thoughts. The fact that Neo's experience of reality turns out to be an illusion doesn't make Neo himself disappear. He continues to exist as the one who has been deceived. The same goes for Descartes. Even if he is not the author of his thoughts, the thoughts still exist in him and he must, therefore, exist. Having concluded that, in order for the thoughts he is having to exist, he too must exist, Descartes then asks what kind of existence this is. His conclusion is that he exists as a thinking thing. That is the most that he can be certain of. His body may be an illusion. Even the particular thoughts he is having may be illusory. But the fact that he is having thoughts remains. This is most commonly summed up in his Latin phrase: *cogito ergo sum*. This phrase, which doesn't actually occur in the book but comes later in his responses to criticisms of the book, is usually translated as *I think, therefore I am*. It arguably translates slightly better as *I am thinking, therefore I am*. The advantage of this latter translation is that it keeps the emphasis on an activity, i.e. thinking.

Descartes then moves on in the subsequent chapters, or days, of the *Meditations* to consider the existence of God, the necessity of free will, mathematical truth and finally the distinction between the body and the mind. While he has doubted everything at the beginning, it appears that his own existence as a thinking thing is not actually the only thing of which he can be certain, although it is the first. He can also demonstrate with certainty that God exists. As he, Descartes, is imperfect, he could not himself create the idea of a perfect being such as God. Therefore, God, as a perfect being, must exist. The existence of God allows him to demonstrate the necessity of free will. As God is perfect, he cannot make a mistake. As we humans are not perfect, we can make mistakes. To make a mistake entails the ability to choose one way or another. This is free will. He also shows that certain mathematical truths are certain. Regardless of experience, the angles of a triangle, for example, always add up to 180°. This is what we might call an analytic truth and, beyond what we would normally conceive of as maths, lends some support to the primacy of logic or reason.

It is, however, the demonstration of himself as a thinking thing which has become the most famous and influential of Descartes's ideas. Where, as we have seen, Luther shifted the conceptual place of man in relation to God and Copernicus and Galileo shifted the conceptual place of the Earth in relation to the sun, Descartes established man as the conceptual and absolute centre of his own world. Or, to be more precise, Descartes established himself as the absolute centre of his own world. Descartes's *Meditations* are written in the first person, as a first-person account of a thought experiment that he is conducting. Strictly speaking, then, his arguments and conclusions only really apply to him. Descartes establishes that he is a thinking thing. He doesn't establish that you are a thinking thing. In order to establish this, you would yourself have to work along through his ideas with him, engaging in the same thought experiment and drawing the same conclusions for yourself. It seems many did, for Descartes' ideas on the *cogito* became so influential that they really come to stand in for the common-sense conception of what it is to be a person. When we think about what we are, even now, we are most often thinking in a Cartesian way.

What Descartes's argument gives us is not just certainty in our existence. If we follow Descartes's thinking, what we arrive at is a view of human existence which is primarily rational. To many people, Descartes's ideas can seem a bit bonkers. Who really feels a need to question everything they know, everything they are and everything they believe? Who really troubles themselves trying to distinguish between dreaming and reality? In that sense, they don't seem that rational at all. But they are rational in the sense that they rely on logic, rather than experience, as their ground. Descartes ruthlessly dispenses with all the givens and rebuilds a world based purely on what he takes to be rational thought. It is, therefore, a strongly rational system of philosophy, as opposed to an empiricist system of philosophy, which would ground itself in experience and the physical world. Within Descartes's system then, the human is essentially rational. Which is to say, we are not essentially physical. Or essentially irrational.

The conception of human being that Descartes gives us has come to be known as the cogito, after his Latin phrase *cogito ergo sum*. It is not only a strictly rational entity; it is also an irreducible entity. This irreducibility is known as atomism. The word atomism comes from the ancient Greek *atomon*, meaning indivisible or uncuttable.

Many Greek philosophers were concerned with understanding what reality was made up of. If you break the world down into bits, you should eventually get to the fundamental building blocks of the universe, the bits that can't be further divided, i.e., atoms. You can see then how Descartes was engaged in a similar enterprise. The key difference here is that Descartes's focus turned to the thinker and the act of thinking rather than the stuff of the world. We might say it turned inward rather than outward. Remember, Descartes titles his book *Meditations on First Philosophy*. He is, therefore, positing the *cogito* or core self as the necessary, or logical, starting point for all other philosophical thinking. The self comes first.

This idea gained considerable traction in European philosophy and was famously developed by Immanuel Kant. Between Descartes and Kant, the cogito can be understood to be a, if not the, core idea of European philosophy. In the English-speaking world, Descartes arguably has slightly less influence and philosophers there have tended more towards empiricism, the idea that the starting point for everything is the physical world. Curiously, these two radically different starting points end up in a rather similar place.

The English philosopher John Locke, who is credited with coining the term 'consciousness,' famously posits that the mind is a *tabula rasa*, a blank slate. What Locke is saying here is that we are born knowing nothing and that all our ideas and understandings of the world come from outside of us. Locke doesn't doubt the world in the way Descartes does, but, these very significant differences aside, he ends up in a strikingly similar place insofar as, like Descartes, he posits the idea of the individual as the centre of all that goes on. Given that the two big philosophical movements of the time, rationalism and empiricism, both kind of agree that the individual is the centre, we can see that this idea has enormous purchase. Whether from a Cartesian or Lockean starting point, the idea is carried forward through political ideologies like liberal democracy, which champions the place of the individual, and the academic discipline of psychology, which predicates its entire field on the notion of the individual. The legacy of the *cogito* remains today, most likely because of some of these fervent champions. It has become a rather common-sense position.

It is not, however, a position which was accepted by everyone. Georg Hegel, who was writing in the late 18th and early 19th centuries, some 200 years after Descartes, contested this conclusion that the self is at the start and conceptual centre of everything. Pushing against both Descartes and Locke, Hegel argued that the self emerges in relation to other people. It cannot, therefore, be understood as the starting point. It is always secondary to the encounter with another. This idea is probably most famously conveyed in what is often referred to as 'the master-slave dialectic.' The passage in question is from a chapter from Hegel's magnum opus, *The Phenomenology of Mind* or *The Phenomenology of Spirit* (depending on how you translate the German *geist*). The chapter is called 'Self-consciousness,' and the relevant section is called 'Of Lordship and Bondage.'

Hegel's basic point is that we require the presence of another to ignite the possibility of our full consciousness. The way Hegel tells it, we have something like an animal consciousness and we seek the recognition of another to allow us to establish a full consciousness (or what Hegel calls 'self-consciousness' – but he is not talking about that feeling of not quite looking right in your new jeans). Key to this movement, then, is desire. Before anything else, we desire something from the other.

The problem, as Hegel unfurls it, is that this transaction is not a straightforward and happy one. The encounter between these two Neanderthal beings is not resolved in mutual recognition. In order to achieve real recognition, you need to be recognised by someone who is in a position to give you recognition. There is no real value in being recognised by someone that you don't value or don't value in the way that you want to be valued. I may gain a certain amount of recognition from my cat, but, lovely as she is, she is a cat, not a person. If I somehow manage to successfully install a new radiator, I may gain plaudits from my non-plumber friends, but given that they are not plumbers and have no real insight into the difficulty or ease of installing a radiator, their recognition doesn't really carry the weight I require. Having endured the sweat, frustration and ultimate success of the, for me, unfamiliar task, what I desire is recognition from someone who really understands the process and pain I have been through. In Hegel's story, it is something a little more profound than domestic plumbing that is at stake, but the principle is the same.

The proto-human wanders the savannah looking for someone who will give him the recognition that he requires. But the someone he finds is similarly looking for recognition. If either of the proto-humans gives the other recognition, then they are putting themselves in a subordinate position. The result, according to Hegel, is a battle to the death, as each struggles to subordinate the other through force.

We can imagine that this scenario plays out a number of times, with one party battering the other to death. The problem with a battle to death is that if it reaches its conclusion, then there is no one left alive to provide the sought-after recognition. It is only in the situation where the defeated party realises that they are about to die, stops and begs for their life, that fought for recognition can be achieved. Except, even here, there is a problem. The defeated one is now enslaved by the victor. They do recognise the victor, as victor or, now, as master. But the problem is that, from the master's perspective, all they have achieved is what we might call slavish recognition. It doesn't carry the value they would have wanted.

Nonetheless something has happened. The establishment of the relation of master and slave institutes a change, what we might call a social change. A new form of society emerges on this basis. Hegel's story goes on, with the slave being put to work and eventually achieving a more substantial form of self-consciousness than the master, due to their confrontation with death and their engagement with the world. But really, for our purposes here, a few things are key. First, the fact that self-recognition, or self-knowledge, emerges through an engagement with another and the fact that the basis of this engagement isn't harmonious but is coloured by aggression, competition and threat.

CHAPTER SUMMARY

In this chapter, we have explored some of the philosophical background for Lacan's thinking. The key ideas covered include the following:

- Augustine and the idea of a narrated life.
- Aquinas and the influence of Aristotle on European thought.
- Descartes and the idea of the individual as an indivisible entity at the centre of their own world.
- Locke and the idea of consciousness and the mind as originally a blank slate.
- Hegel and the notion that our idea of ourselves emerges through an encounter with another.

4

THE MIRROR STAGE

Lacan takes the basis of Hegel's story and applies it to his understanding of contemporary existence. Like the proto-human of the Hegelian myth, Lacan argues, each of us starts out seeking recognition, or seeking love. One of the key insights, which is implied rather declared, in Hegel's text is the idea that desire is what motivates our encounter with the other. Or, to put this in a slightly different way, in Lacan's version, our encounter with the other occurs simultaneously with the emergence of desire.

Lacan has a famous saying that "desire is desire of the Other" (Lacan, 1977: 312). This is one of these statements which can, and indeed really must, be read in a number of different ways. We can understand Lacan as saying that the primary (meaning key and first) thing we desire is another person, usually our mum. At the same time, he is saying that desire is something we learn from others. We model both the manner in which we desire and the things that we desire on the way we see others desiring. You can see this function in celebrity endorsements of consumer products or in product placement in films. A dress is desirable because Margot Robbie wears it on the red carpet. A car is cool because Ryan Reynolds drives it. We even desire Margot Robbie and Ryan Reynolds because they are presented in such a way that we understand them as being desired by other people.

Desire is also the desire of the other, in that we want to be wanted by the Other. Whether this Other is embodied in our mum or Ryan Reynolds (and it is rarely, if ever, straightforwardly singular), we desire their desire. And in this wanting to be wanted, we can also recognise a base sociality. Few of us are truly happy without other people there, at least some of the time.

DOI: 10.4324/9781315622002-4

This notion of desire as being at the base of what we understand ourselves to be can be understood to be the basis of Lacan's idea of the mirror stage. Importantly for Lacan, however, one of the others we encounter at this formative level is our self or perhaps better said – for reasons that will soon, hopefully, become clear – our idea of our self.

Lacan tells how as an infant we each encounter our image in a mirror and experience a combination of jubilation, disappointment, anticipation and antagonism. Importantly, for Lacan's argument, the human infant is born premature. Unlike foals, for example, we don't start to walk minutes after birth. Human babies can't generally even hold their own heads up until they are about four months old. They only start to walk at around six to eighteen months, and will generally initially do so with the aid of a walker or some sort of trolley to lean on. That is to say, they initially require a prosthetic device to allow them to move around. All this emphasises a profound state of physical dependence which marks the human child apart from the rest of the animal kingdom. As the child's awareness is developing despite its dependence, this gives rise to a sense of its own incapacity or inability. The child can't walk, but it can see other people walking.

Babies aren't very coordinated, seemingly unable to control their own arms and legs terribly well, and yet they see others who appear to be more coherent. Lacan argues that this gives rise to a disjunction between what the child sees and what it experiences. This disjunction is carried through to its own encounter with itself in the mirror. When the baby is held up to a mirror – remember, it can't yet do this itself – it sees what looks like a coherent entity. Its arms and legs are joined to its torso, with its head sat on top. It looks whole. And yet, the child's everyday experience of itself is less connected. Without the visual distance the mirror provides, the everyday experience of one's own body is less immediately coherent and this is, we might assume, even more the case with a baby, who lacks the abstract idea of what a human body should be onto which to map their experience. Anyone who has ever had a filling will know the experience of suddenly not being able to tell where their lips are. Or if you have ever sat in one position too long and numbed your own leg, only to stand up and stumble.

Added to this, when we look in a mirror, the image we see reflected back at us is distorted and necessarily only partial. Especially those in the US or Canada will be familiar with the safety message on car wing mirrors saying, "objects in the mirror are closer than they appear." Mirrors tend to enlarge the image reflected. They also invert the image. Who hasn't been puzzled by a photograph where a distinguishing feature appears to be on the wrong side of their face? We are used to seeing ourselves the 'wrong way round' and then take the photograph – which arguably presents a more accurate version, or, at least, is closer to the version that other people see – as somehow wrong or even disturbing. Finally, the mirror, rather obviously, only presents the surface and, even then, only (usually) the front surface of the body and, most often, only the top part. Our experience of ourselves is complex – in the proper sense of the word 'complex' – bringing together numerous different elements. We have moods, we have thoughts and we have hunger pangs, pains and grumblings. These experiences are not reflected in the mirror, or not directly. The back of our head is just as much a part of our physical body as the front of our head, but it is rarely something we see in the mirror, except at the hairdressers and is not usually what we think of when we think of ourselves.

What all of this adds up to is that the mirror image is really very different from the immediate experience one has of oneself. In the case of the infant, we can imagine that this distinction is perhaps more pronounced, insofar as the infant lacks the comprehension or understanding that would allow an adult to grasp, process and manage the differences. An adult might look in the mirror while experiencing indigestion and not be concerned that the reflected image doesn't reflect the discomfort they are experiencing. An infant, we can imagine, might be more affected by this distinction. That said, even adults might, at some level, be perplexed or even distressed by the mismatch between the mirror image and their own experience or idea of themselves. Think of cases of body dysmorphia, anorexia or depression. In the case of the infant though, the experience, Lacan argues, is formative. As the infant has no prior or given idea of themselves, their formative encounters, which work to build their idea of themselves, are not based on a simple correspondence between what they see and what they feel. Rather, they are built on a disjuncture, on a mismatch between image and bodily experience and, importantly, on the reinforcement from others that this image *is* them. What the infant sees, and what the infant is told is them, doesn't fully correspond with what they experience. Or we might say that it doesn't correspond at all. One is an image, apparently coherent. The other is a complex of incomprehensible sensations, emotions and confusions. If we accept this description, this formative mismatch, then we need to follow through on its ramifications.

Lacan describes this mismatch as an experience of *méconnaissance*. This term is usually translated as misrecognition, in the sense that we misrecognise the mirror image as our self. We could say, we mistake it as our self. We take it in and assume it as the basis of the idea of who or what we are, even though it is clearly not who or what we really are. It is an external, partial and distorted reflection of light. *Méconnaissance* also has a suggestion of knowledge (*connaissance* in French), so it is knowledge which is formed on a mistaken basis. And, breaking it down further, *naissance* is birth, so it is the origin of our idea of our self. Putting these various connotations together, we can see the richness of Lacan's choice of term in *méconnaissance*. It conveys an idea of an origin based on mistaken knowledge.

A crucial point here, when we talk of mistakes, is not to be lured into the idea that because this idea of what we are is mistaken, there is another, better, more accurate idea available. Our cultures are full of ideas of true selves, and much of the industry of self-help or therapy is based on the idea that, beyond the false or unhealthy notions we have of ourselves, there is a true inner self waiting to be uncovered. We talk of finding ourselves, of getting back to ourselves, of not feeling ourselves and of being authentic. Lacan is pushing against these notions and positing a considerably less comforting idea that behind the mistaken idea of our self that we glean from the mirror, there is nothing else. Or put slightly differently, the idea we glean from the mirror is the basis of our identity and there is nothing more primary which precedes this.

It is perhaps useful to recall the full title of the short article on the mirror stage Lacan published in 1949. Its full title is 'The Mirror Stage as Formative of the *I* Function as Revealed in Psychoanalytic Experience.' While perhaps not very catchy, the full title does spell out much of what is at stake here. The I, the sense of I, of identity or personhood, is described as a function, not a substantive entity. We should remember that Freud, the inventor of psychoanalysis, described the psyche as being composed of three elements: the ego, the id and the superego. The term ego, which has become rather commonplace in English, is actually the Latin word that James Strachey chose to translate the German word *Ich*. *Ich* simply means I. So, when Lacan talks of the 'function of the I,' he can be understood to be talking of the ego, and he can be understood to be specifically talking about the ego that can be seen in the clinical setting, how it shows itself through the analysand's speech.

In differentiating the ego (or I) from the id and the superego, Freud was, of course, already making the point that our sense of identity, our sense of who or what we are, was only ever partial. We are, in Freud's theory, just as much our id and superego as we are our ego. Like ego, id is a Latin word; this time it was Strachey's choice of translation for the German *Es*, meaning 'it.' The 'it' refers to that part of us which is untamed or not under our control. Freud famously compares the id to a wild horse, with the ego as the rider. A horse is much more powerful than its rider would be and the rider has, nonetheless, to constantly keep the horse in check. Freud believed that we live in this constant kind of inner tension. The id is only really interested in pleasure, and immediate pleasure at that. If we succumb to the id, we may have a great time, but it would likely turn into a bad time before too long. Think of Sam Levinson's HBO series *Euphoria*, where the teenage characters appear to do little but party, but nobody actually seems to be having a very good time at all. Freud's point is that the id may want to drink, gorge, fuck and sleep, but if we were just id, we would soon die. We need the ego to make plans, to achieve balance or moderation. We need the ego to tame the horse.

The third aspect of the psyche, the superego, relates to this as it is our internalisation of the rules of society, usually the rules we take from our parents. We might think of this as our moral side, but it is not necessarily so in a way that is as positive as that initially sounds. The superego can be cruel, making us feel guilty and causing inner conflict as we, paradoxically, derive pleasure by depriving ourselves of pleasure. Such is the complexity of the self.

Returning to Lacan, then, we can see that his focus at this point is primarily on one aspect of the Freudian self: the ego. This is the dimension of the self with which we most readily identify, and it is really this process of identification that Lacan is interested in here. By identifying with our mirror image, we start to build an idea of our self and this then grows and solidifies as further identifications confirm or extend earlier identifications. But because this identification is based on something external, there is a fundamental flaw in this operation. We have taken in what is essentially an alien idea – something strange, foreign, something other. This alien invader appears to be more coherent and together than we are. This alien other doesn't have our unhappinesses, our pains, our confusions. It isn't disjointed and uncoordinated. This doesn't only mean that it doesn't fit with our experience in and of our body, that there is a mismatch. It also, according to Lacan, creates a three-way dynamic. First, as we have seen, it sets up an identification, however flawed or misled that identification may be. But precisely because it is flawed, it sets up an antagonism, a rivalry. This alien other that I have introjected is better – more complete, more whole, more capable – than I am. Now, to feel an antagonism or aggression towards an external other is one thing, but when that external other is internalised and taken to be your self, then the aggression is necessarily also turned towards yourself.

More positively, the perceived distance between the image and experience creates what Lacan calls an anticipation. I may not be that coherent, complete object I see in the mirror, but I might start to believe that I could one day be that.

In the interplay of this identification, antagonism and anticipation, we can see the influence of Hegel and, most especially, the centrality of the notion of desire. It is, Lacan is telling us, precisely through what we are not, what we are lacking, that we come to experience desire and this desire is primarily a desire for what will make us whole.

CHAPTER SUMMARY

In this chapter, we have explored the basic ideas of Lacan's theory of the mirror stage. The key ideas covered were:

- The fact that desire is something we learn, both in terms of its form and content.
- That we develop an idea of ourselves based on an encounter with an external image.

- The contrast between our experience and our idea of ourself gives rise to a mismatch and creates a sense of lack.
- There is no correct or true version of oneself behind or beneath one's mistaken idea of oneself.
- The self is not a coherent singular thing.
- The process of identity formation entails lack, aggression and anticipation.

5

IMAGINARY/SYMBOLIC/REAL

We have seen how, in the mirror stage, an ambivalent antagonism is established between the child and its mirror image. A question that is often raised here is, what if the child is blind? A completely blind child would not be able to see their image in a mirror. Would this mean that they simply wouldn't develop in the way that Lacan describes? A first thing to perhaps emphasise here is that Lacan isn't really talking about a developmental stage at all. Yes, he makes a great deal of discussing our premature status at birth and the baby being held before a mirror, but really, he is describing an ongoing process of always failing identification which affects adults just as much as it affects infants. The mirror as physical object, and the particular experience of looking at your own image in a mirror, is only one way of capturing, or experiencing, this process. The same effects could easily be imagined with a child's encounter with a teddy bear. In reality, a child doesn't only have one experience, and nobody is for a moment suggesting that your idea of your self erupts from a single encounter. Along with mirrors and toys, children necessarily experience other people and these other people are a continuing element of identification. This is clearly not only the case for children, and while the visual element might often dominate, it is not exclusive. The other we experience in the mirror, then, is one other which forms an important basis of identification, difference, anticipation and antagonism, but it is not the only one. Other others, other people, such as siblings, parents, friends, neighbours, pets, toys, cartoon characters, etc. all function in the process of identification and continue to do so throughout our lives.

DOI: 10.4324/9781315622002-5

This process of identification, formed through our encounter with these various others, constitutes one important dimension of how we experience the world. Lacan argues that our experiences of the world can be understood to be configured through three distinct modes. He calls this first mode the imaginary. We usually think of imaginary as meaning made up or not real. Children often have imaginary friends, characters they have invented, whom they talk to but whom only they can see. In a sense, this is close to the idea of the imaginary that Lacan is discussing but with the important proviso that, where a child's imaginary friend is understood to not actually exist and can be contrasted with their friends in reality, this contrast doesn't apply in Lacan's usage. For Lacan, all of the child's friends are, to an extent, imaginary. Moreover, the key imaginary friend a child has is the child themself.

As we have seen in the discussion of the mirror stage, the child builds up a sense of itself, an idea, drawn from its external encounters. This allows the child to create an identity, and it is this imagined identity which is both the fruit and the basis of the imaginary realm or, we might say, the imaginary dimension of our experience of the world.

When I say it is both the fruit and the basis, I am pointing to the perpetual circularity of the experience. Our idea of our self is based on a minimal recognition of or identification with an external body or image. From this, we start to build further elements of identification and this process continues throughout our lives. Importantly, for Lacan, there is no determinable starting point for this process. The process could only be understood as potential once it is underway, so any starting point could only be projected backwards and is, therefore, always, itself, imagined.

This imagined identity then forms the basis of our relationships with our self and with others. It can be understood as the basis for group identities, friendships and preferences of all sorts.

It is also, however, never fixed. We might imagine the infant as an unformed discontinuity which is given some form by the mirror encounter, but this form is only ever partial and never entirely fixed. It is a little like a prosthetic encasement which holds the child together. In this sense, the shape the child takes on is more the shape of the casement than the shape of the child, but the child comes to assume that this shape is itself. The casement can be altered and ongoing, new experiences will affect the becoming adult's identity. Overall, however, the more this assumed identity is reinforced, the less it is likely to change, and then the more it is likely to be reinforced, but always with an irreducible sense of misfitting, because the imagined identity is not actually who you are.

We have focused on the straightforward scenario of the child in front of the mirror confronting a gap between, on the one hand, its own immediate experience of its body, its emotions, its sensations, its thoughts and, on the other, the seemingly coherent mirror image. We can understand that there is necessarily a gap there, a gap between what is and what might be. Let's now broaden out to the wider context of the child's coming to grasp a(n always incomplete) sense of itself.

The mirror image conveys the physical dimension or, better said, as an image, it conveys the imaginary dimension. A child's growing sense of what it is, however, is also carried through the language that surrounds it. Parents talk to and about their children from the very beginning. Long before a child is even conceived, the people who will become the parents will have expressed ideas of who their child will be. When the child is in the womb, the parents will discuss it, talk to it and read to it. The very moment a child is born, it is born into a room literally full of people talking about it. As the child grows, this world of words surrounds its every moment. Even when there are no people talking, the words will have started to go into the child and will soon start to come out of the child. We start then, without ever really having to think about it, to formulate ideas of what and who we are. Sometimes we are told directly who or what we are – good boy, clever girl, naughty child, etc. At other times, we take in an idea of who or what we are because of what is not said, for example when one sibling is praised for some accomplishment or behaviour and the other is not. The early ideas about the not yet born, or not yet even conceived, child may have seemed like an idle fancy to the not yet parents, but these ideas can take root and continue to resonate through the now living child's life. General ideas of children, formulated long before the child's birth, will come to effect how the specific child is expected to fit into the world. While the notion that boys should be attired in blue and girls in pink might seem old fashioned now, similar such preconceptions continue to circulate and often without us being particularly aware. Parents and grandparents often seem compelled to make comparisons – *he's so like his father*, or *oh, you used to suck your thumb in exactly the same way*.

There are three conceptually related things which we need to draw out of this, and an important, conjoined, conclusion which follows. The first point is that thought is constrained by language. The second that the child is born into language. The third that the child's sense of itself will, at the very least, be heavily influenced by what is said about it. What these three points lead to is an unavoidable sense of alienation.

Let's begin with point one. Language is the stuff of thought. Without language, we may experience the world and we may have sensations and feelings, but it is only with language that we are able to represent these, combine them and invent new ideas. Now, if we consider that there are only so many words available and that any one language follows certain conventions, or ways of talking about things, not to mention the grammar through which the language operates, then it becomes clear that the ideas we have – about the world, but also about ourselves – are conditioned by the language(s) we have learned. This is not to say that we cannot combine words in new and interesting ways or even, as Lacan himself does, create new words. But even these moments of creation must be harnessed to the already existing language or they would appear as mere gobbledegook or noise. The poetry of Edward Lear, often referred to as nonsense poetry, is a good example here. Lear creates new words, but he combines them with known words and inserts them within conventional grammatical patterns. Take his most famous poem, *The Owl and the Pussy-cat*. After running away and getting married, the owl and the pussy-cat "dined on mince, and slices of quince, / Which they ate with a runcible spoon" (Lear, 2014). There is in fact no such thing as a runcible spoon, but it is clear that the word runcible, despite not existing and having no meaning, is an adjective.

Not only are we limited by the form of language, but the very world we live in – our way of thinking about it – is largely determined by our language. In English, we talk of a leg, meaning the body part extending from our groin to our ankle. In some Chinese dialects, a single term, *jiǎo*, is used to include both leg and foot. Physically, speakers of English and speakers of Chinese are more or less built the same, but the way their languages organise their bodies is starkly different. Similarly, you have probably all heard the cliché, popularised by Kate Bush, about the Inuit having 50 words for snow. There is some debate as to how true this really is, although in some Inuit languages there are numerous different words for snow, in part because they are agglutinating languages (meaning that, where in English we would add an adjective, for example, in these Inuit languages they add to the word itself). This gives rise to more words for snow than we have in English. Beyond this, we can understand that in a land where snow is more plentiful and more of an everyday concern, people are likely to have more complex ways of talking about it and distinguishing between different types. The broad point here is that what we think, however original it might be, is constrained in numerous ways by the language in which we think it.

A pertinent final example here is that given by the German philosopher, Friedrich Nietzsche. Commenting on the idea of the cogito we discussed in Chapter 3, Nietzsche points out that Descartes's conclusion is more of an effect of language than anything else. *Cogito ergo sum*, as we know, is commonly translated as *I think, therefore I am*. While in Latin, the *I think* is formed by a single word (*cogito*), it still contains the idea of *I*. *You think* would be *cogitas*, *he thinks* would be *cogitat*. Nietzsche's point, which is a bit clearer in English, is that when I say 'I think, therefore I am,' I have already presumed the 'I' in the first part of the sentence, only to then conclude that it must exist in the second part. It is a faulty logic, but one which is an effect of language. It isn't possible to formulate the sentence in Latin without assigning a (grammatical) subject to the action. Similarly, in English, we say 'it's raining,' but it isn't very obvious who or what is doing the raining ... maybe the sky? God? Because our language doesn't readily allow a formulation which doesn't contain a grammatical subject, we end up thinking the activity, in reality, must imply a subject in the philosophical sense, i.e., an actor, someone who or something which does the doing.

The second point that we need to draw out here is that none of us invented the language that we speak. It, quite literally, was around before we were. This has the effect that the child arrives into and has to learn to express its ideas in a medium that is not its own. All the ideas we have of the world, the very ability to process the world in thought, is conducted using a toolkit which was made by others. This then extends to the thoughts that we have about ourselves. All our ideas of ourselves, our most intimate thoughts, our dreams or aspirations, our reflections and our conception of what we are, all of these are necessarily formulated in and through a language which comes from outside us and which preceded us.

Thirdly, linked to the previous point, as ideas about the child will have been formed before the child is born and expressed repeatedly after it is born, the child cannot but ingest these ideas. That is to say, all the things a child hears about itself, even, or especially, when it isn't really aware that it is hearing them, or doesn't remember hearing them, will go in. It is not even necessarily a case of the child hearing the ideas expressed. Ideas circulate and affect behaviour, including behaviours which affect the child or shape the environment into which the child must enter.

The obvious example here is stereotypes or received notions of wider groups to which we are supposed to belong (whether we actually choose to belong to them or not). This would include ideas about gender, nationality, religious affiliation, race and class. The fact that we don't necessarily or actively choose membership of these groups doesn't stop us becoming members of these groups, and the fact that we aren't actually born with the attributes associated with membership of these groups doesn't stop us beginning to exhibit these attributes. Nobody, male or female, is actually born with a natural propensity to play with construction vehicles (simply because construction vehicles are not, themselves, natural things). Even less obviously constructed (excuse the pun) characteristics are impossible to discern on an absolute scale. Are women really more nurturing than men? All of them? All of the time? This is not the place for a debate on gender attributes or nature versus nurture, the point is rather that these ideas circulate and their very circulation has effects. If everyone ingests the idea that girls are more compliant, a lot of girls are going to find themselves falling into this pattern of behaviour, and those that don't are likely to find themselves being labelled differently because they don't.

Closer to home, and bundled in with these social stereotypes, children grow up hearing descriptions of themselves, suggestions of what they like or are like, comparisons with others, half-heard judgements and innocuous comments. These all add together to create impressions which are impossible for the child not to take in. The sheer volume of comments a child will hear means that the 'message' is rarely going to be straightforward, but the point remains that a picture is built up that has its source outside of the child and outside of any particular person's consciously formulated idea of what the child is, will or ought to be.

What these three points, brought together, lead us to is the fact that what we come to think of as our self – our personality, our likes, our dislikes, our strengths, our failings, our desires – is derived from the outside. Which is to say, it is not us. This places something of a contradiction at the heart of our sense of identity. That which is most me in me, isn't in fact, or isn't originally, me at all. And, if we recall one of the key points from the mirror stage, there is not another, alternative, truer version of me waiting to be excavated from beneath this. But the lack of a truer version doesn't stop us hankering for one.

Lacan explains this mismatch in our sense of self in terms of a movement from being to meaning. If we accept the idea that we are immersed in a world of language, that language colours and shapes how we process and conceive everything in our world, including ourselves, then, in accepting this point, we are still potentially left with a sense that there is a possibility of a clean or pure access to the world, one which is free of the power of language. Many people do hold to this idea, and many will have found the suggestion that we live inescapably in language quite objectionable or even ridiculous. People often recourse at this point to moments in nature – a sunrise, the night sky, mountains, scuba-diving, sex – as if these experiences, by mere dint of the fact that they occur, in some sense, apart from social life or culture, can be held up as examples of experiences beyond language. But if we think about it, our experience of the night sky, even our understanding that the night sky is the night sky, never mind our understanding of planets and stars and the stories of the constellations, are all formed and brought to us through language. The awe we feel beneath the night sky is expressed in language. The same goes for all these examples. We may feel we lose ourselves to the experience but in order for the experience to be recalled, even seconds later, as an experience, it has to be formulated in language, even if we are only formulating it for ourselves.

The idea of a world untainted by language is, we might say, a fantasy. It is in many ways a comforting fantasy. We might even say that it goes to the core of what the term fantasy means in psychoanalytic theory, but we will come to that.

As well as holding on to the idea that there is a world we can access without or beyond language, people will often harbour the idea that there must have been an experience of the world before language. Now, in some senses, we can see how this would be true. Putting aside the fact, discussed above, that babies are in language long before they can produce language, and even before they are born, most of us would accept that young babies are not capable of using language. Babies, of course, have brain activity and sensations. They do have needs and make demands. It would be a stretch, however, to say that they think. Accepting this idea would be to place babies in a world before language, at least in terms of their ability to utilise language to organise their experiences of the world around them.

Even if we do accept this picture, there is necessarily a marked difference between the experience of being a thinking, language using human being and the experience of being a non-language using baby. Moreover, this difference isn't a simple us and them difference, where only a baby can grasp what it means to be a baby and only a non-baby can grasp what it means to be a non-baby (we are including here not only adults but also children once they have learned to speak). Nor is it the case that the non-baby could somehow recall the baby experience and simultaneously hold both that and their later, language infused experience. The difference is lopsided in that only the non-baby has the ability to conceive anything at all, as it is only once we have language that we are capable of formulating coherent thoughts.

So, on the one side, we have an experience which cannot be conceived (although we can imagine that it might, or even must, have taken place), and then on the other side, we have the experience of being in language. Put simply, the very ability to think the experience of being outside of language can only take place inside of language. The idea of being without language is an impossible idea, not in the sense that it can't have happened, but in the sense that it can't be formulated from within.

Putting babies aside for a moment, there is an important point here that carries through our lives as human beings. The idea that we somehow co-exist in being and meaning, that, as we often oddly put it, we have both being and meaning, doesn't work. It doesn't work because the two are mutually exclusive. The odd phraseology, the idea of having being and meaning, is illustrative here in that it suggests that the holder of being and meaning, the one who would have them, is somehow outside of or separate from both.

Lacan uses a colourful analogy to convey his point about this movement from being to meaning. He asks us to imagine a highwayman holding up a stagecoach. When the highwayman cries "stand and deliver, your money or your life!", the choice isn't, in reality, between your money or your life. If you were to choose willingly to give your life, it is improbable that the highwayman is going to leave your money sitting by the side of the road after he has killed you, and, even if he did, it is difficult to conceive in what sense it would still be your money. You would be dead. The choice is, at best, forced. Even, on the other hand, if you were, as you most probably would, to choose to sacrifice your money, there is a high chance that you would be left for dead anyway.

Lacan's point here is that the apparent choice between being and meaning is similarly impossible. Were we to (impossibly) choose being, it would be literally inconceivable in that we would have no concept of being to choose and no deliberative powers through which to choose it. It is only from within the world of meaning that any choice can be made at all. The very notion of an existence prior to (or outside of) meaning is something that can only be posited from within meaning. The choice of being is, then, an unavailable choice.

This realm of meaning is what Lacan calls the symbolic. We might think of it as the partner of the imaginary. Where the imaginary describes our modes and processes of identification, the symbolic describes the structures in place which give our world meaning or order. We have focused on language as a key element of this, but it also encompasses all the other structures or systems which govern our ability to make sense of the world and function together within it. While the imaginary necessarily involves other people, it has as its focus, or tether point, the subject. We might then say that it is the more subjective dimension of experience. The symbolic, as it is concerned with language and law and systems, is the more social dimension. As we've noted above, language always precedes us. The same is clearly true of laws, society and social systems.

You will often read people referring to another Lacanian concept, the big Other, or just the Other (always with a capital O). The capital O here distinguishes the Other from the other, in the sense of other person. The big Other is often used in a way that makes it sound like a synonym of the symbolic order and to some extent this is true. To some extent, but not exactly. The simple way to think of this is that the symbolic order refers to the abstract notion of the interlocking systems of rules that govern our experiences of the world: language, law, conventions, morality, road signs, financial exchanges, etc. The symbolic order is the impersonal fact of the system of rules and the structure of rule that frames, limits and governs our experience of the world, including our experience of ourselves. The big Other, on the other hand, is the subjective encounter with this symbolic order.

There is a curious story told by the Priest in Franz Kafka's *The Trial* about a man from the country who finds himself before the door of the law. He waits there to be let in, and he waits and waits. In fact, he ends up waiting his entire life, and as he is about to pass away, he asks the doorkeeper why it is that all the time he has been waiting, no one else has ever come by. If this is the door to the law, surely it must be the door for everyone. That, after all, would be our understanding of the law, that it is neutral and applies equally to everyone. No, says the doorkeeper, no one has come by because this door exists only for you. The point is that, while the law may, at least in principle, be applicable to everyone, the application is necessarily always singular. Or, put slightly differently, the law as an edifice may exist as a singular idea, but when we encounter the law, that encounter is necessarily specific to each of us. The same is true of the symbolic, and it can be understood to manifest in two related but distinct ways.

First, there are different languages in the world and each of them existed before each of us, but our particular encounter with language, our vocabulary, the particular sense we take from words and our expressions are all particular to us. In this way, we can begin to see how the symbolic and the imaginary necessarily work together. When I hear or read something, I am interacting with the symbolic dimension. The sequences of words are governed by certain rules, and the words are associated with certain definitions. The definition of any word requires more words. Think of how you use a dictionary.

You aren't sure of the meaning of a word, you look it up in the dictionary, which takes you to more words. What the dictionary doesn't provide you with, however, is the particular associations the word carries for you. Think of the word dog. This might conjure the image of a dog for you, but it is going to conjure a different dog for each of us depending on our particular experiences.

Second, as we each have our own particular understandings or particular configurations of associations and experiences, we also then experience a certain otherness to the symbolic order. There is, so to speak, a gap between you and the symbolic order, and this manifests as a sense of exclusion. The world seems to be working in a certain way, but I am not really sure what that way is. I'm not sure how I am supposed to fit into the world. I am not sure what it wants of me.

We might call this a personalisation of the symbolic order. I associate the structures and rules that are the symbolic order with other people, as well as with apparently human systems. I personalise the impersonal by imagining knowing operators behind the curtain managing and orchestrating things. It doesn't really matter if it is God or the Wizard of Oz or the Rothschilds. The point is that I posit someone or something as the knowing operator. In this sense, then, the big Other can be understood as the individual's experience of the symbolic order, but it is then the symbolic order connecting to the imaginary order.

Lacan argues that the two orders – the symbolic and the imaginary – are necessarily bound together. They rely on each other, not just in terms of our positing of the big Other but also more generally. There is, however, no totalisation here. Combining the symbolic and the imaginary doesn't explain everything in the world and doesn't capture everything about every experience we have of the world. It is impossible, in any one situation, to ever say it all. There is always something missing. This is not simply a matter of always being able to add to any description or account with more detail, in an endless accumulation of words. It is also the case that there are always, so to speak, gaps in the words we produce. The particular structure and makeup of any one language is such that it necessarily excludes as it includes. A pertinent example of this would be the categories of male and female. By partitioning living entities into two groups, we necessarily exclude anything which doesn't fit into these two groups. We simply, at least for a long time, didn't have any words for those that didn't fit the binary positions available. Vague terms like 'intersex' function more as a catch-all synonym for 'not included' than they do describe a substantial category of their own.

Of course, we can create new words to describe new categories, entities, activities or ideas, and we can keep adding new words infinitely. But that is rather the point, no matter how many new words we add, we would never have exhausted the potential of human experience.

Adding new words is also not always as straightforward a solution as we might want to believe. Again, the example of gender identities is a good case in point. While we might have, at least in part, become more accepting of the possibility of more than two gender identity positions, we are still a long way from having achieved clear and universally adopted terminology for additional positions.

The same kind of point can be made in relation to the quantum developments in physics in the 20th century. Scientists like Werner Heisenberg confronted aspects of the existing explanations of the physical world which didn't cohere, breaking entirely new ground and necessarily producing new ideas which are still confounding for most people now. We can understand that what Heisenberg and his colleagues achieved was an unsettling of the symbolic order, predicated on the fact that, neat as it appeared to be, the existing knowledge didn't actually explain or account for everything. We might say that Heisenberg confronted a reality beyond the known world, not in the sense of an intergalactic exploration, but precisely in the sense of contemplating the gaps in the structure we have erected to explain the world. That is to say, the gaps in the symbolic.

Lacan calls this unknown dimension the real. If we were restricted to the imaginary and symbolic, to our points of identification and the structuration which makes much of life possible, we would, arguably, be completely contained. There would be nothing more to say, as it would already have been said, and nothing more to experience. Life in a purely symbolic realm would be a little like a dynamic death. We might move around, like pieces in an elaborate mechanism, but we would have no volition, no real choices to make. We wouldn't really be alive in anything but a biological sense of the term. Adding in the imaginary dimension in a sense does little to alter this picture, other than to give us a lens through which to believe that our movements around the mechanism are meaningful.

This picture is a little like the Wachowski's film *The Matrix* that we discussed in relation to Descartes's questioning whether he was dreaming. Before we get to the character of Neo in the film, we meet Thomas Anderson, the character of Neo before he, and we, discovers the matrix. Thomas is a computer programmer, living a mundane life, working in an impersonal cubicle in an open-plan office, much like a mouse in a maze. Everything in Thomas's life is predictable. He is trapped in the symbolic universe. It is only in his out-of-work, online life, as a hacker that he at least entertains the idea of something more than the symbolic trap. Here, he encounters the idea of the Matrix, and, shortly afterwards, he is arrested and experiences an inexplicable series of events which he can only rationalise by assuming he dreamt them. That is to say, they were imaginary.

He is later informed that these nightmarish events were not a dream, and is then offered an explanation. The explanation he is given is that the world he had assumed to be real was actually a sophisticated fiction. Thomas is really in some kind of dormant state, encased in a pod which is plugged into an AI network which has effectively enslaved humanity and is powering itself off their bio-electric energy. If we take, in terms of our analogy, this network to be representative of the symbolic order, and the identity and personal experience within this fake reality to be representative of the imaginary, then we could say that the new world with which Thomas is confronted, the reality of pods and AI masters, is the real.

Where this analogy breaks down, however, is that the real is ungraspable. The world of the pods, what the character of Morpheus in the film actually refers to as 'the desert of the real,' is, in Lacanian terms, simply another version of the symbolic. A true Lacanian version of *The Matrix* would entail an endless series of levels of reality, each another variation of the symbolic, with the realm of the real never evident. Or, we might say that the most Lacanian part of the film is the beginning, when Thomas experiences the mundanity of his alienated life but also experiences something within that that he cannot put his finger on, something pressing that he cannot account for, the fact that the supposedly all-encompassing structure of reality is not actually all encompassing at all.

For Lacan, it is the insistence on the real that offers the possibility of a truly subjective engagement with the world. Without the real, all is preset. The real is not, however, something we could occupy. To live, we have to live in the symbolic and imaginary, with the real always imposing. To capture this idea, Lacan makes use of a curious configuration of circles called the Borromean knot.

A Borromean knot is a little like a Russian wedding ring, with three interlocked bands. The crucial difference is the way in which the bands are locked together. If you were to cut one of the bands in a Russian wedding ring, the other two would remain connected. In the case of a Borromean knot, each band is interwoven with the others in such a way that severing any one band would cause the other two to also separate. You can try this at home yourself with some rubber bands (Figure 5.1).

Lacan's point in his recourse to the knot is that the imaginary, symbolic and real are not merely three modes of experiencing the world or three different mechanisms which facilitate different aspects of human experience. Rather, the three realms or modes are necessarily always operating together. Each moment we experience partakes of imaginary, symbolic and real elements, inseparable

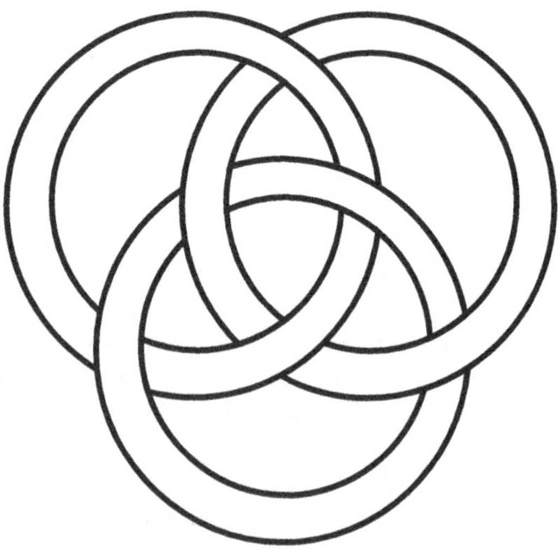

Figure 5.1 The knotting of the realms of the symbolic, the imaginary and the real.

from each other. If we were to separate them, our experience of what we take to be reality would fall apart, as happens in cases of psychosis.

CHAPTER SUMMARY

This chapter sought to outline Lacan's tripartite idea of the imaginary, the symbolic and the real. The key ideas it covered were:

- Identity is an always ongoing process of identification. Our identifications shape our relationship with the world and others in the world. Lacan calls this mode of experience the imaginary.
- We are born into a world of language and other systems of rules. These structures govern our experience of the world. Lacan calls this mode of experience the symbolic. The fact that language is always alien to us, but a primary means by which we know or think of ourselves, means that we are always alienated from ourselves.
- Although processes of identification and the fact of language allow us to process and relate to the world, they are necessarily incomplete modes of experience. There is always something beyond our identifications and beyond our abilities to articulate our experiences of the world. Lacan calls this beyond the real.
- These three modes of experiencing the world are bound together in a peculiar knot which is structured in such a way that cutting any one of the rings will result in the other two also becoming detached from each other.

6

OBJET PETIT a

When he presents the Borromean knot as an illustration of the knotting together of the imaginary, the symbolic and the real, Lacan places a small letter *a* in the very centre. This *a* refers to one of the most widely known concepts from Lacan's work, what he calls *objet petit a*. These days writers on Lacan usually leave this term untranslated, although you will encounter it rendered slightly differently in different texts. *Objet* is the French for 'object,' and is, like the English, used to refer to both everyday objects and the specific psychoanalytic idea of an object (i.e., the object of affective or sexual energy), as well as forming the opposite of the idea of the subject. The term subject is one commonly used in philosophy to refer to the abstract notion of a person. It is also, in French *(subjet)*, an alternative term for the analysand or the psychoanalytic patient or client. The *petit a*, little a, simply indicates the lower-case letter *a*. Originally, this *a* was a reference to the small initial letter of *autre*, meaning 'other.' So *objet petit a* might be rendered 'object little o.'

When Lacan talks about the *autre* (other), he is talking about other people but particularly in the sense of those that are other to you. That is to say, the term quietly evokes the idea of the subject and places an emphasis on difference. By taking this notion and converting it into a particular piece of terminology, Lacan is working to distinguish the concept from any particular application of it. That is to say, while the *a* of *objet petit a* might have originally indicated the other, as in other person, by distilling it to a single letter, Lacan is turning it into something like an algebraic unit, like the x and y you will have encountered in maths class. The point of these algebraic units is that they don't have any value of their own but function as

DOI: 10.4324/9781315622002-6

placeholders for a value. They also don't have any meaning, in the sense that they aren't apples or oranges or dollars or metres. They are voids. Lacan's *a* is the same.

An important aspect of this is that, aware of the tendency we have to form identifications, to make connections on an imaginary level, Lacan was keen to do what he could to stop those he taught (or those who later read him) from falling into this imaginary lure. Utilising a pre-existing word (say, for example, *autre*) would have unwittingly been encouraging people to not only limit their understanding to that one understanding of the term but would also have been unwittingly encouraging people to make their own personal connections and associations with the term. The simple lower-case *a* has a much more neutral appearance and, arguably, does achieve something of this value- and meaning-free status. Arguably, though, nothing really escapes this lure, and we will still tend towards particular usages of *objet petit a,* and particular examples do tend to circulate and dominate. It is, as we saw in the previous chapter, impossible to ever truly escape the imaginary.

As mentioned above, the idea of an object in the field of psychoanalysis has a specific denotation. In our formative and ongoing encounters with other people, we generate certain ideas. These ideas serve to provide a certain sense of stability or consistency. While, of course, your mother is a complex, multifaceted person, with many likes, dislikes, moods and even appearances, who will behave or speak differently in different contexts and with different people, it is necessary to distil a coherent sense of her in order to be able to recognise and relate to her. Just as, in Lacan's theory of the mirror stage, the idea we have of our self isn't true, as such, so the idea we have of other people is never – could never be – true. People are far too complex and varied for that to be the case. As we cannot grasp the whole complexity of, for example, our mothers, and we couldn't really function very well without some recognition of them, what we internalise is a version of them. Freud called this version an object. Put simply, then, an object, psychoanalytically speaking, is our internal version of the people in our lives.

When Lacan talks about *objet petit a,* then, he is referring to other people, but not other people in their own unique individuality and separate lives. Rather, he is talking about other people as they are for you. The version of these other people that you relate to, however contestable that version may be from some supposedly objective perspective.

This underscores an important point here. From a psychoanalytic point of view, there is no objective perspective. Or, perhaps better said, the idea of an objective perspective is irrelevant. This is largely a statement about the nature of psychoanalytic practice and the clinic. If an analysand is talking to their analyst about something that their husband said, it really doesn't matter if the account is empirically accurate, if that is actually what he said, if it supposedly happened in reality or in a dream or, indeed, if the analysand is actually married at all. What matters is the effect this supposed encounter or conversation had upon them. From a more philosophical perspective, there is also the base point that it would be impossible to ever actually establish an objective truth in these kinds of situations. All we have to go on, and all the analyst is interested in, is the analysand's version.

Lacan's use of the term *objet petit a* dates from 1957, but the idea he is conveying through it is already evident in the *Mirror Stage* essay. He goes on to use a number of different terms to convey a similar, although not necessarily identical, idea, drawing attention to what we might understand as different aspects of the concept. These other terms include *das Ding* (from the German, meaning the Thing), *lathouse* (an untranslatable neologism which we might roughly render as little thingamabob), *agalma* (literally meaning a statue, but in Lacan's use referring to that mysterious or ineffable something in someone that ignites or sustains our desire) and surplus enjoyment (a term derived from Marx's theory of surplus value and referring to our imagining of the pleasure that others enjoy and we don't). *Objet petit a* is also often referred to as the object of desire or the object cause of desire.

When we think of an object of desire, we usually think of a physical thing that we want, perhaps a luxury item, maybe an esteemed work of art. If you google the term, you are likely to find lots of references to a 1977 film by the Spanish film director Luis Buñuel, *That Obscure Object of Desire*. Buñuel's film concerns one man, Mathieu, and his lifelong infatuation – or, we might say, desire for – a young woman, Conchita. Buñuel, as a surrealist, was interested in psychoanalysis and the exploration of dreams and the unconscious, as is immediately evident in many of his films. That *That Obscure Object of Desire* is told through a series of flashbacks itself echoes the dynamic of a psychoanalytic session. The idea of the object of desire as another person isn't that unusual, but it is worth emphasising here that the person as object in Buñuel's film is strikingly close to the sense of object in psychoanalysis outlined above. This is underscored by two specific points from the film. First, the character of Conchita is played in the film by two different actresses, and not in a sequential manner but interchangeably. Second, Mathieu's desire for Conchita is never consummated.

The use of two actresses could be understood to illustrate the specifically psychoanalytic sense of object; that it is an internalisation or version of the person rather than the person in themselves. It also, within this, draws our attention to the fact that the person as an object is never consistent or is never self-identical. Now, common sense would suggest that if there is one thing with which someone or something ought to be identical, it is their self. That is kind of what the word 'identical' means. Two things are identical if they are the same, if they share the same identity. It seems a bit nonsensical to suggest that something could not share in its own identity. Nonetheless, this is what psychoanalysis suggests. We should recall the problematic of identity in the mirror stage, the fact that identity is something which comes, not from birth, but from a later encounter with an external world and is assumed on the basis of an image from that external world which never quite fits with our own experience of ourselves. This gives some sense to the idea that we, and people in general, might not be self-identical.

The use of two actresses might also be understood to point to the fact that the thing which is desired is never actually that thing we encounter in reality. As mentioned above, in 1960, Lacan used the Greek term *agalma*, from Plato's *Symposium*, to refer broadly to the idea more commonly referred to as *objet petit a*. The *Symposium* largely concerns the idea of love, and the term agalma is used by the character of Alcibiades to refer to that indiscernible or hidden aspect or element of someone that causes you to fall in love with them. That *je ne sais quoi.* If we keep this idea in mind, we can begin to separate the person, in an everyday sense, from that thing that we can't quite put our finger on that keeps us infatuated, that keeps our desire alive. This links then with the second point; that Mathieu's desire for Conchita is never consummated.

If we are really thirsty, we might find ourselves a large glass of cold water and quench our thirst. We then stop being thirsty. If we are hungry, we eat and our hunger is abated. If we are cold, we can put on a jumper. If we are tired, we sleep. In each of these cases, something is missing, and by finding that missing something, we, so to speak, fill the gap. Lacan calls this gap need.

Need is generally biological or body based. We need to eat, sleep, drink, etc. We can see these needs very clearly in babies. It is generally what makes them cry. Once provided with the thing that will satisfy the need, the baby stops crying.

What is interesting in the case of babies, however, is that the satisfaction of these basic needs is almost always accompanied by attention, affection and love. When a baby is hungry, the mother (usually) will feed it, and this will involve skin-on-skin contact, the soothing warmth of breast milk (or heated formula), a cuddle and a feeling of safety. It is understandable then that the baby will start to make an association here between the arrival of the food-stuff that will satisfy its need and the arrival of love. It is likely then that the baby will form an attachment to this loving feeling and then begin to cry not only when it is hungry, tired or uncomfortable, but because it wants love.

Lacan distinguishes this second lack from need and calls it demand. Where the focus in need is on the stuff that will satisfy the need – if you are really hungry, it doesn't really matter who brings you food, it is the arrival of food that matters – the focus in demand is on the other person and, specifically, on the love. Whatever we demand, Lacan is saying, beneath the proclaimed thing we are demanding, it is a demand for love. When you ask your friend or your teacher to help you with your assignment, it may well be that you really need some help with your assignment but, bundled up in this, it is quite likely that you also, or especially, want some attention, company and love.

Desire is set apart from these two other modes of wanting. Desire, for Lacan, is always a desire for *objet petit a*. Need can be, albeit temporarily, satisfied. If you're hungry, you eat a sandwich, and you stop being hungry. Of course, you will get hungry again, but you can eat something else and you will stop being hungry again. In the case of demand, you want love, and you get some attention and affection – manifestations or indications of love – but it isn't like a sandwich. It may go some way to making you feel better, but it doesn't fill the gap in the same obvious way that food satisfies hunger. Desire is one step further along in this step towards impossibility. Desire, in Lacan's understanding, is never satisfied.

This can seem a little pessimistic or fatalistic. If desire can never be satisfied, then what is the point? The point, we might argue, is precisely that it is never satisfied. Flipping this around the other way, if desire were to be satisfied, then what would we do afterwards? A perpetually unsatisfied desire is precisely what keeps us keeping on. It is, we might say, the engine of life. Desire, in some way, shape or form, is what gets us up in the morning, what motivates us to study, pursue a career, write a book, climb a mountain, learn an instrument, have sex, form a relationship or have kids. But none of these things, as pleasing or satisfying as they might be, actually exhausts our desire. Once you achieve the grades you aspire to achieve at school, your attention moves on to, for example, university. Once you have earned your degree, you may choose to undertake another or get a job. Once you have landed your dream job, you will want to move up in the ranks, start your own business or simply earn more money. Very few people who write a book or a song, or paint, only write one book or one song, or paint one picture. Fewer people only have sex once. While you may only get married once, or only have one child, these are by definition incomplete desires in that a relationship develops and requires constant attention, a child grows and our desires become desires for our children to succeed, blossom and be happy. The point is that desire is endless and this endlessness is the movement of life. This doesn't, of course, stop the endlessness of desire from also being extremely frustrating.

Objet petit a, then, might be understood as the conceptual stand-in for all these other things that we want, the mathematical placeholder which we can deploy in our theoretical conjectures to understand desire in an abstract manner. Lacan's idea is, however, in a sense, quite the opposite. For Lacan, all these other things are the stand-in for *objet petit a*. Each empirical or even abstract (if we think of love or happiness, for example) thing that we desire is, Lacan argues, a substitute for *objet petit a*. And because they are substitutes for the *objet petit a*, attaining them never really scratches that itch.

In the 1980s, the Coca-Cola Company ran a successful and catchy advertising campaign with the tagline "Coke is it!" (1984). There was never any explanation as to what 'it' was, but that was just the point. Coke, apparently, was the answer, the ultimate satisfaction. It was it. Except, of course, it wasn't. The paradox of the advert was that the sugar content of coke makes you thirsty, so drinking it makes you want more of it. Like all the other stand-ins for *objet petit a*, coke isn't it at all and having grasped (or drunk) it, because it isn't it, your desire remains unsatisfied.

But what then is this mysterious *objet petit a* that lies behind all the things we think we want? It is, Lacan says, the object cause of desire. It is that which makes us desire. And what is this? Quite simply, it is the existence of lack.

A useful metaphor for *objet petit a* is perhaps a black hole. A black hole is an unobservable entity. The force of gravity in or from a black hole is so strong that nothing escapes it, including light. What can be observed of a black hole, then, is an absence and, importantly, its effects on other entities. We can, theoretically, circle a black hole, but we can never grasp it as such. The intensity of the gravitational pull of a black hole not only ensures that nothing escapes from it, but it also exerts an unrelenting and irresistible attraction. It sucks everything that is remotely close to it, into it. It is in these senses that we might say that *objet petit a* can be compared to a black hole. Like a black hole, it is undetectable, other than as an absence. That is to say, *objet petit a* is undetectable in itself, but discernible through its effects. And, one of those effects is its unfailing pull. *Objet petit a*, then, describes a gap, an absence, a lack. But it is a productive lack, in that it continues to have enormous effects.

Freud's theory suggests that, from birth, we experience a series of losses which leave us marked and forever searching to re-establish a lost unity or bond. *In utero*, the child is linked to its mother by the umbilical cord, and they are, then, in a sense, one. After birth, the child is no longer physically attached to the mother, but remains largely attached. Freud places particular emphasis on the breast at this stage. A breast-fed baby latches onto, quite literally attaches itself to, the mother's breast. Unlike the experience in the womb where the conjoining was consistent and all engulfing, the breast-fed child will sometimes be on the breast and sometimes not. Sometimes the breast will be there, sometimes it will not. Sometimes it will be forcefully removed. The initial separation or loss of mother-child unity which comes with birth is then followed by an instability, with the object of satisfaction manifesting as inconsistent. Children are eventually weaned, and the inconsistency is resolved in a fuller loss.

There is, however, an ambiguity to each of these stages. The *in utero* unity is arguably not a unity at all. Yes, the foetus and the mother may be biologically conjoined, but the very fact that we would conceive of them as conjoined or linked suggests that we conceive of them as two, and not one. We would generally accept that, umbilical cord notwithstanding, there are two distinct entities. After being born, the on/off relationship with the breast itself already suggests an ambiguity, and this carries through to the relationship with the mother more generally as the child grows.

The point is that there are losses or feelings of loss, but these are also bound up with strivings for control, recognition or independence.

We should also keep in mind the idea from the previous chapter that the movement from being to meaning is one which is only conceivable from a position of meaning. That is to say, the movement from being to meaning can only ever be retroactively posited. The simple idea of a lost unity appears then to be a supposition.

Lacan suggests that the actual source of lack, the feeling of having lost something, arises from elsewhere. We have seen how in the mirror stage experience the infant is confronted with an image supposed to be itself but that it is an image which appears to be more coherent and complete than it experiences itself to be. We have also seen how we are each born into a world of language which is fundamentally alien. This alien language into which we have no choice but to be born, however alien it might be, is the only means at our disposal to formulate an idea of our self. There is no true you before the idea of you that you take from the mirror and from the language in which you are expressed. You are then stuck in an impossible position of being an alien to yourself, of being alienated. Bringing these ideas together, Lacan argues that the human subject is necessarily split. We are split between being and meaning. We are split between our experiences of ourselves and our ideas of ourselves. We are split by the sheer inability of language to capture everything and our inability to capture anything without language.

Another way that Lacan expresses this is to say that we are barred. We might think of this in the sense that one is barred from a nightclub. We are not allowed access to ourselves. We're not allowed in. The bar also indicates a division, a classic Freudian division about which we have said very little so far, between the conscious and the unconscious.

This chapter sought to outline Lacan's concept of *objet petit a*. The key ideas covered were:

- An object in classic psychoanalysis is our mental representation of another person
- *Objet petit a* is not actually an object at all, it is the gap that we seek to fill with other objects, either in the sense of people or in the sense of things, or the absent thing that will complete us.
- The urge to find this something that will fill the gap or incompleteness we feel is what Lacan calls desire
- Desire can be distinguished from other wants, namely need and demand.
- Desire is never actually satisfied
- Desire can be understood as coterminous with lack
- The lack that we experience is rooted in a series of impossibilities and disconnects:

  - the impossibility of language expressing everything
  - the fact that we can only conceive of ourselves in terms which are fundamentally alien to ourselves
  - the fact that the basis of our never-ending process of identification is a misrecognition of an external object as ourself
  - the split between the unconscious and the conscious mind

7

THE UNCONSCIOUS

Freud is usually credited with the invention or discovery of the unconscious, but the concept has a slightly longer history. The German term *Unbewusste* is used in 1800 by the philosopher Friedrich Schelling in his book *System of Transcendental Idealism* and then shortly after in English by the poet Samuel Taylor Coleridge in his autobiography. Schelling's use of the term notwithstanding, Freud makes the point, in his 1923 book *The Ego and the Id*, that when philosophers talk about the mind or thought, they are almost always talking about the conscious mind or conscious thought. Freud's point here is that philosophers, who study and explore questions of human thinking and existence, have a tendency to miss a big part of our thinking and being. An illustrative example of this is Descartes's *Meditations*, when he arrives at the conclusion that the one thing of which he can be certain is the fact that he is thinking. As Descartes 'thinking' here is his own active process of doubting what he can know, his thinking is very much conscious thinking. He even kind of acknowledges this himself and extends his probing doubt to ask what happens when he is not thinking. We might retort that on the level of biological brain activity, we are always thinking, but this isn't what Descartes means. When he says thinking, he means thinking of which he is aware. Conscious thought. Descartes rightly acknowledges that there are moments when we are not aware of our thinking. We can undoubtedly all relate to this. Who hasn't lost themselves in an activity to the point where they are unaware of what they have been doing? And, of course, we sleep. This gap in conscious thinking is a bit of a problem for Descartes. His whole

DOI: 10.4324/9781315622002-7

certainty of his existence is predicated on the fact that he is thinking. If he is not thinking, then how can he be sure he still exists?

His neat solution to this is God. As God, according to Descartes, would not deceive, He can function as the guarantor of the continuity of existence in the gaps between the moments of thinking. Another solution to this problem might simply be the unconscious.

Freud uses the term unconscious in two related but importantly distinct ways. As an adjective, the term simply designates those thoughts or elements of thoughts of which we are not conscious. For example, we say, in this sense, that I unwittingly called my friend the banker a wanker because I had an unconscious urge to put him down. Freud also, however, uses the term as a noun, referring to an apparent substantive entity called the unconscious.

In his early work, in what is referred to as his first topography (his first model of the mind), Freud argues that the mind can be thought of as consisting of three parts: the conscious, the preconscious and the unconscious. The preconscious refers to the knowledge and memories – the thoughts – that we have freely available to us. If I now write the word hippopotamus, it is unlikely (though not impossible) that you were already thinking about a hippopotamus before you read the word, but when you did read the word, you can easily bring to mind a hippopotamus. It may be a hippopotamus you once saw at the zoo, a favourite soft toy, a character from a children's book or simply some hippopotami that you saw on a natural history programme. The point is, you not only know what a hippopotamus is, but you can conjure up particular hippopotami from memory. If I asked you to remember the last time you saw a naked adult, you could probably, similarly, easily recall the occasion, whether it was yourself in the mirror, a partner or perhaps an image or a character from a film.

These memories or bits of knowledge reside in what Freud called the preconscious. When you recall them, they are brought into consciousness.

Consciousness itself is, according to Freud, a fleeting moment. Nothing really resides for long in the conscious, simply because our attention is constantly being drawn on to new things. Our consciousness needs to be conscious of what is going on around us. Our consciousness needs to concentrate. As you read these words, you are, hopefully, conscious of them and the explanations I am trying to present. You may be less conscious of what else is going on in the room because few of us can focus our conscious attention on multiple things.

Now, you were presumably able to recall the last naked adult you saw without too much effort. It presumably wasn't that long ago. If I asked you now to recall the first naked adult you saw, few of you would be able to do so with such surety. In fact, I would guess that none of you would be able to do it all. One simple explanation for this might be that someone who is an adult now would first have seen a naked adult many years ago, when they were a child. Most of us would have seen our parents in some state of undress when we were very young. We don't remember this, presumably precisely because we were very young and it was a relatively long time ago. While this explanation might make some sense – our ability to recall things does fade over time – it isn't really terribly convincing. While it is true that we forget things, or lose details, over time, this fading isn't entirely uniform. Now, we might argue that we remember those things which are important for us to remember, but then we also, frustratingly, forget many things which are apparently important. Freud suggested something else was going on here.

The basis of Freud's idea of the unconscious is that we repress difficult, challenging, conflicting or simply unpleasant memories or thoughts. He argues that it is a basic mode of self-preservation. We can make an equation here between the child taking in experiences and the child, as most do, putting things in its mouth.

Young children often put all sorts of things in their mouths, sucking them and then discarding them or swallowing them. We might assume that the basic mechanism here is pleasure and displeasure. If the thing put into the mouth tastes good, or feels nice, the child is likely to keep putting it in its mouth, or perhaps swallow it. If the thing tastes bad, or hurts, the child is likely to expel it. And possibly cry.

Freud's hypothesis is that something very similar goes on with thoughts or experiences. If a child sees, hears or experiences something pleasant, they would be likely to revisit it. They might revisit it by re-experiencing it and doing whatever they had done again. They may revisit it by recalling it, bringing it back to mind and experiencing it mentally. If, on the other hand, the experience was unpleasant or painful, in some sense threatening or frightening, then the child would want to expel the idea, in much the same ways as they would expel a foul-tasting olive they had mistaken for a sweet grape. The problem is that you can't simply spit a thought out.

Repression is the solution to this, the next best thing to spitting out a bad-tasting thought. Repression is the expelling of the thought from conscious or preconscious thought into the unconscious where it can no longer be easily recalled. There is, however, an obvious difference between the expelled food and the expelled thought. The expelled food is out of you, gone. The expelled thought isn't. It is only out of the consciousness-preconsciousness.

Freud argued that those memories or thoughts which have been repressed have a natural buoyancy, a tendency to resurface. As they have been consigned to the unconscious, they can't very well simply re-emerge. The force of repression works to keep them down. Instead, they seek to re-emerge by attaching themselves to related ideas or memories or manifesting through physical symptoms.

Freud's famous published cases all offer different examples of this mechanism at work. It is worth remembering that Freud was a practising psychoanalyst or therapist. He didn't come up with the idea of the unconscious in isolation but rather arrived at it in an attempt to explain his patients' behaviours, symptoms or peculiar ways of suffering. As a medical doctor, Freud's first route to explanation would always have been the obvious physical explanation. If a patient was experiencing a persistent cough, Freud would look to discern whether there was an infection or injury causing the cough. If the patient was experiencing paralysis of their arm, for example, he would attempt to rule out physical injury or nerve damage. Only after ruling out physical causes would Freud look for mental causes. At other times, the problems his clients were enduring were more immediately obviously mental or behavioural rather than physical. A patient might be overwhelmed by an inexplicable fear, a phobia. They have found themselves stuck in a repeated and harmful pattern of behaviour. Essentially, Freud, through his work with people who were suffering in some way, discovered that there was something apparently inexplicable at work, something which didn't lend itself to easy resolution through existing diagnoses or explanations. The idea of the unconscious is not, then, simply an abstract theoretical construct. It emerges as a gap in our understanding of ourselves.

A lot of the language utilised here, in the discussion above, seems to give the impression that the unconscious is a space or an aspect of us, almost as though it is a physical thing. I recall a student once complaining that they 'physically couldn't understand Lacan' and one of my colleagues, slightly cruelly, retorting, 'you should try using your mind.' The point here is that the mind, and thus the unconscious, are not meant to designate a physical part of us. Nonetheless, we do tend to speak of the mind and thoughts as something 'in our heads,' which is, of course, a physical thing. The picture can, therefore, quite understandably get a bit confusing. It is important to try to keep this separation in mind though. The unconscious, despite the metaphors of basements, attics or storerooms which are often used, is not actually a space or an empirical entity. Repressed thoughts are not physically stored somewhere. They aren't actually pushed down. They don't then actually float up or find their way out. These are all just ways of speaking. Ways of speaking which can sometimes end up being a bit misleading.

This is perhaps one reason that Freud moved away from his conscious/preconscious/unconscious model as a way of theorising the operations of the human psyche. The physical metaphor seems to imply that the unconscious is a singular part of us and that there is a neat divide, almost like a wall or a lockable door, between one part and another. In his later work, Freud developed a second model that focuses on what we might call psychic mechanisms or agents: the ego, the id and the superego (see Chapter 4). The term unconscious then begins to have more of an adjectival usage as each of the psychic mechanisms, we might say, partakes of unconscious forces.

In his early years, Lacan tended towards this adjectival use of the term unconscious. When he starts to employ the term as a noun, it is in a substantially different way from Freud.

Psychoanalysis, as we have seen from the beginning of this book, is and always has been concerned with language. The basic fact of psychoanalysis is two people in an isolated and one-sided conversation. Nowadays, more and more people are experiencing psychoanalysis over Zoom or by telephone, but this doesn't affect the fundamental dynamic which constitutes psychoanalysis. Traditionally, the two people would be in the same room, one lying on a couch or chaise-longue, the other sitting in a chair behind them. The analyst would be behind the analysand so that they, the analysand, couldn't see them. This set-up is usually recreated with long-distance or tele-analysis. What this set-up allows, then, is the foregrounding of the speech which takes place, which is to say, the foregrounding of the language produced.

In recognising this centrality of language, not just to analytic experience, but to human experience generally, but especially to analytic experience, Lacan places language and how language operates at the core of his theory. It is often commented that Freud developed his ideas of psychoanalysis before the emergence of the academic field of structural linguistics. Lacan is the one who brings the two fields together. We have already seen, in the discussions in Chapter 5, how the fact of language and our experience of the world through language structures how we conceive of ourselves and our relation to the world in which we find ourselves. Let's now look at language itself and how it operates in a little more detail.

The Swiss linguist Ferdinand de Saussure is generally considered to be the father of structural linguistics. Saussure argued that language should be thought of as being made up of two basic components, what he called the signifier and the signified. The signifier is what we would in common terms call a word (although it might also be a phrase as, in terms of meaning production, there isn't really any significant difference). This signifier can take the form of a written word, a spoken word or even a thought word. The signifier is really the idea of the word that sits behind any particular instance of the word. So whether I say either, or you say either, regardless of our particular accents, we are both utilising the same signifier. If we weren't, we wouldn't be able to understand each other. The signified is the counterpart of the signifier. It is the idea or concept that the signifier seeks to convey. Importantly, for Saussure, the signified isn't the thing in the world. It is the idea. So if you say tomato, it conjures an idea of a tomato for me. There doesn't need to be an actual tomato present. This is important for Saussure because it underscores the fact that language is a coherent system, not simply a mechanism for pointing at things in the world.

Saussure then argues that the signifier and the signified are bound together.

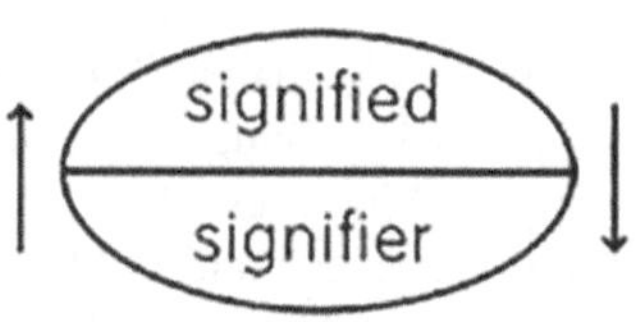

The production of the signifier, through speaking or writing, produces the signified for the listener or reader (and, of course, for the speaker and writer too). The two are welded together. A signifier which had no attached signified would not be a signifier, it would be a noise or a squiggle. A signified with no signifier is not even conceivable.

This is not, however, to suggest that there is necessarily an exclusive one-on-one relationship between the two. A word can quite easily have two meanings. The words bear and bare sound exactly the same but have quite distinct meanings. Moreover, the word bear in itself has two distinct meanings, such that a bear may bear something on its back while at the same time being bare naked.

Added to this, we don't actually communicate by producing isolated signifiers. Signifiers always exist in relation to each other. They do this in two aspects. When we communicate, we do so in a sequence. Whether we are writing or speaking, one word follows another. The order in which the words follow each other produces certain meanings, but this order is also largely determined by the rules or grammar of the language we are speaking.

In English, a sentence usually requires a subject and predicate; the someone or something that is the key focus of the sentence and something about them or what they are doing. The predicate always needs to include a verb, a word which indicates the action or state of the subject. It may also include an additional bit of information, such as descriptive words, or words indicating position or relation. It will often also contain a second someone or something who sits in relation to the subject, connected by the verb. We call this the object. *I love Atticus* includes *I* (the subject) doing the loving (verb) to or about *Atticus* (the object).

While in English there is some flexibility to the word order (what we call syntax), this is limited. If you mess with the order too much your speech becomes incoherent or just sounds ridiculous, or like Yoda.

Saussure calls this unfolding sequence of words the syntagmatic axis. The structures of our language work to render this axis as limiting or partially predictable. If you produce the beginning of a sentence, I don't necessarily know in advance what the end of the sentence is going to be but the possibilities are not unlimited. If you say *Peter kicks* … with a combination of grammatical knowledge and familiarity with how or in what contexts those words tend to be used, I can make a reasonable prediction that the sentence continues … *the ball*. Or it might continue … *Jane* or … *the bucket*.

There are certain words or phrases, sequences of signifiers, which could fit and certain that couldn't.

It is also uncertain, particularly in speech, when the sequence has ended. *Peter kicks the ball* could become *Peter kicks the ball so hard that it breaks the window*. And on and on. Saussure calls the choices of words which might fit into the sequence at any one juncture the paradigmatic axis. We can think of this as follows:

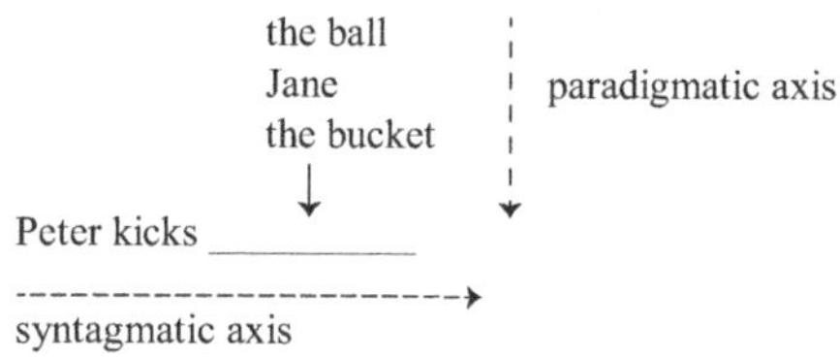

Each choice from the paradigmatic axis closes down or modifies the available choices for what follows on the syntagmatic axis, and the populated syntagmatic axis, in turn, closes down or determines the available options which would constitute the paradigmatic axis.

Saussure's insights (and we have only glossed the very basics here) helped Lacan to think how the subject relates to and through language. This constitutes a very important, influential and far-reaching aspect of his development of Freud's theory, one which affects how he thinks of the subject and, then, necessarily, how he thinks of the unconscious.

Going back to the basic idea of the signifier and the signified, Lacan takes this seemingly simple observation and develops it to its logical conclusion and the ramifications that spill from this. The signifier and the signified are wedded to each other, but only one side of this pairing is observable. We speak or write words and we then hear or read words. The signifier is this overt aspect of language. It is always, however, accompanied by an invisible, indiscernible but utterly necessary side, the signified. Without the signified, there is no language, just noise and scribbles. But this essential element always remains unseen or unheard. Unseen and unheard but evident in its impact nonetheless. Sticks and stones, they say, can break your bones, but names will never hurt you. But they are wrong. Words have very profound effects on us and they do so because they signify. This evident but invisible dimension of language echoes a formulation Freud had used many years before.

In his first great book, *The Interpretation of Dreams*, Freud writes about dreams having both manifest and latent content. This is, in part, the point Lacan is picking up in relation to language. Like dreams, everyday speech has something like manifest content and latent content: the signifier and the signified.

In the same book, Freud discusses other aspects of how dreams work, key amongst which are displacement and condensation. Displacement refers to the process whereby one idea is shifted onto a somehow related idea. We often, in dreams, appear to displace our feelings about one person onto another. You might dream of Spiderman, when actually you are concerned with something to do with your father, who happens to be called Peter (for those who don't follow Marvel, Spiderman's name is Peter Parker). Here, one idea, Spiderman, is substituted for another idea that shares some of its properties (in this case the name Peter). Displacement can also take the form of one idea being replaced by an idea not so much due to the sharing of properties, but more because the two ideas are habitually associated or one is a generally thought of as a part of the other. You may dream that you are fishing when your concern is actually your grandfather with whom you spent significant moments fishing as a child. You may dream of a particular skateboard that appears to make no sense until you remember that a friend you lost had a similar skateboard.

What each of these examples illustrates, in Freudian theory, is that an idea can be replaced by another idea. In terms of understanding repression, the point is that the repressed idea is, as a repressed idea, by definition, too difficult or unpleasant to manage. By displacing the core of the idea from one representative onto another, what was repressed is able to make itself known, albeit in a rather cryptic fashion. Or, in Saussurean terms, we might say, one signified is replaced by another, while the signifier remains the same.

Condensation works by a similar logic. In condensation, a number of ideas are merged into one representative. Imagine you dream of your boyfriend, but he is dressed and is acting like your father. Your dream has condensed the idea of two people into one to convey a single notion.

By drawing on the insights of structural linguistics, Lacan allows us to appreciate that these mechanisms aren't restricted to the work of dreams but are functioning all the time in the language we speak when we are awake. In part, this can be understood in terms of Saussure's syntagmatic and paradigmatic axes. As the sentences we produce unfold along the syntagmatic axis, we are constantly selecting terms from the paradigmatic axis to add, to continue the sentence or speech or writing. This also operates receptively, as we listen or read we are constantly predicting what will come next, as each addition adds to or changes the potential meaning of the sentences we are, for example, hearing.

This doesn't necessarily mean that we are in a constant state of suspense. There are points at which we reach a meaning, where sense appears to be anchored. Even then, however, the potential meaning can, and often will, open up again.

Lacan calls these anchoring points *points de capiton*, after the French term for the buttons used by upholsterers. The function of these buttons in upholstery is to stop the stuffing in a cushion or chair from moving around. The *point de capiton* does the same for meaning.

A classic example of this is The Who's song *My Generation*. When Roger Daltry sings "Why don't you just …" and then performatively stutters the next word, repeating the 'f' sound. The effect is that the listener anticipates what might come next, what signifiers are available in the paradigmatic axis. The obvious one is perhaps 'fuck off,' but this would not have been an acceptable phrase to use in a pop song in 1965. Daltry then fills the gap and sings "fade away," but 'fuck off' hasn't entirely disappeared, despite having never actually been uttered.

This doesn't only manifest in this overtly performative way. Imagine a friend tells you that they are leaving town to embark on some exciting new life adventure. You may be really happy for them, yet, at the same, you may feel less than happy at the idea of them no longer being around. You respond that you feel 'slad,' a condensation of the signifiers 'glad' and 'sad.' I recall once a colleague talking at length, ostensibly about his wedding, and each time he, presumably, meant to say 'wedding,' he said 'funeral.' One idea was displaced onto a connected idea.

We can understand these substitutions and agglomerations in terms of Saussure's paradigmatic axis. In the case of displacement, the (seemingly) wrong signifier is being selected. In the case of condensation, available signifiers are being combined.

The psychoanalytic setting is, as we've said, fundamentally built on the idea of the analysand talking. As an analysand, you are expected to freely associate. What Freud, and subsequent psychoanalysts, mean by this term is that you talk trying as hard as you can to not think consciously about what you are saying. This means ignoring many of the basic rules of conversation that we learn as we grow up. Foregoing these conventions is actually rather hard. Freud's idea was that if we could succeed in freely associating, we would create more opportunities for the unconscious to speak. We are usually conscious of the person we are speaking to and want them to take a certain meaning from what we say, even if, in reality, we can't control what meaning they take. On a very basic level we usually try to make sense. We avoid jumping around, seemingly randomly, between topics. Or at least most of us do. We are often selective in what we say to people, censoring ourselves and holding back embarrassing or shameful ideas or stories or even specific words. Usually, we want to present a certain idea of ourselves. Or, at least, we want to avoid presenting some ideas of ourselves. But however we speak we do present an idea, or lots of ideas, of ourselves.

In the context of the psychoanalytic clinic, then, one could say that all the analysand is doing is presenting, or constructing, an idea of themselves. Whatever the analysand is talking about – their childhood, their parents, their marriage, their dreams, a movie they saw the night before or what they had for dinner – whatever it is they speak about, they are (also) speaking about themselves.

Picking up on this basic insight and combining it with Saussure's model of the signifier and signified, Lacan draws our attention to the fact that the self, or, as he calls it, the subject, is always what is conveyed from one signifier to another. In a sense, you could say we are sustained by our speech. But what is sustained here is something which only exists in this speech. This is not, of course, to say that, as physical entities, we would somehow cease to exist if we stopped speaking. The point is rather like Descartes's thinking thing that can only be certain of its own existence as long as it is thinking. Lacan's point pushes further and focuses on the stuff of thought. We think in language and it is this that maintains us.

Let's try to map out the logic at work here. Language is made up of signifiers – the words and phrases we hear, see, speak and write – and signifieds – the ideas attached to or provoked by the signifiers. Signifiers are always associated with other signifiers, both in the sense of being substitutable for each other and in the sense of predicting each other. It follows then that any utterance will convey or invoke not only a straightforward meaning but will also unwittingly convey or invoke a bunch of other associations too. Keep in mind that the associations are in the language, not in some separate thought process we are having apart from the language. There is no thought process apart from the language. We then hear the unheard in what is said, whether we are aware that we hear it or not. We think the assumption we made about where the sentence was going, whether we are aware that we think it or not. We make this or that association with this or that signifier, whether we are aware that we have made it or not. Or, perhaps better said, the association is made, the sentence opens certain possibilities, and the signifiers resonate.

The obvious objection here might be that, while we may speak the same language as those around us, we don't all have the same vocabularies and we don't all have the same associations with the various words we know. This, however, is rather the point. Rather like the door to the law in Kafka's story, each of us has a unique experience of language. But this doesn't mean that we have access to a unique language. The fundamental structure of language remains the same.

Recall the point we explored in Chapter 5, that language necessarily exists before and outside of each of us. Combining this idea that language is external or fundamentally alien with the insight that you are what is created and conveyed by the signifier you speak, leads Lacan to conclude that we need to reconsider what is meant by the idea of the unconscious.

The sense of the unconscious that many have taken from Freud is that it is an internal function. This seems rather commonsensical. Each of us is a self-contained entity, with our own perception of the world, our thoughts, both conscious and, then, it follows, unconscious. The idea of my unconscious being filled up with repressed thoughts from my past rather fits with this.

The idea of the unconscious had already been a rather provocative idea when Freud floated it. The idea that people were not really in control of themselves, not really in their own driving seats, so to speak, is sometimes referred to as a second Copernican revolution. Copernicus, some years before Galileo, had argued that the Earth wasn't the centre of our solar system, displacing humankind from the physical centre of 'their' universe. Freud's arguments about the unconscious are then an even more devastating blow, as they suggest that I (in terms of my conscious self, or ego) am not even the centre of my own existence. Lacan takes this point one step further and argues that the unconscious is not even individual.

What Lacan is talking about here is not some kind of universal, mythical or shared unconscious. Rather, he is making the somewhat more straightforward point that the unconscious is an effect of language and, as language is not something internal and individual, then neither can the unconscious be. Language is something that exists between us and, thus, it makes much more sense to conceive of the unconscious as something that is produced between, or at least outwith, us. If we take a moment to consider this point, it starts to make some real sense, challenging as it may be to grasp. If thoughts occur in language and I, as an idea I have of myself, am an effect of the language that is produced in relation to me, and this language contains not only the direct or acceptable meaning but also a variety of associations, then it follows that the sentences that I speak (and hear) will contain both the direct message and the associations. This, Lacan argues, is how the unconscious works.

CHAPTER SUMMARY

This chapter outlined Lacan's conception of the unconscious. The key ideas explored were:

- Freud used the term unconscious both as a substantive (i.e., the unconscious) and as an adjective (i.e., describing some idea as being unconscious).
- Freud distinguishes the unconscious from two other elements of the psyche, the conscious and the pre-conscious.
- Freud argued that we repress unpleasant ideas and this is what constitutes the unconscious.
- Lacan reconceived the unconscious, drawing on insights from structural linguistics, particularly Saussure's idea of the signifier/signified pair.
- Developing from this idea, Lacan argued the unconscious is structured like a language.

8

SEXUATION

Up until now, we have talked about the subject or person as a single thing, as though we were all largely the same. This is not, however, the case for Lacan. He makes a number of distinctions which are essential to both the clinical practice of psychoanalysis and to our understanding of how people function (or don't) in society.

First of all, Lacan recognises that there are different sexual positions in society. This is not simply to acknowledge the fact of different reproductive organs nor is it, for Lacan, as simple as acknowledging the fact that we assign different attributes to boys and girls.

Freud, arguably, pinned a lot on basic biological differences, not in the sense that these differences determined who you were so much as that our different bodies gave rise to different points of identification. To be slightly reductive, boys have penises and girls don't. This leads boys to identify with their fathers and girls to identify with their mothers. This process of identification mobilises through what is probably Freud's most famous bit of theory, what he calls the Oedipus Complex. Even now, the basic ideas of the Oedipus Complex are shocking, or distasteful and unacceptable to many.

Freud draws on Sophocles's play, *Oedipus Rex*, which tells the story of the King and Queen of Thebes of whom it is foretold that they will have a son who will kill his father and marry his mother. Disturbed by this prophesy, the King and Queen decide to have the baby killed and charge a soldier with the task of taking the infant to the hills and slaughtering him. The soldier cannot bring himself to do this and instead gives the baby to a shepherd who in turn gives the baby to the childless king and queen of Corinth. Oedipus subsequently grows up in a different royal household, utterly ignorant of his true origins.

DOI: 10.4324/9781315622002-8

Oedipus then visits the oracle himself and learns that he was foretold to kill his father and marry his mother. Shocked by this, and eager to subvert the prediction, Oedipus determines not to return to Corinth. Of course, what he doesn't know is that the king and queen of Corinth are not actually his parents.

On the road to Thebes, Oedipus encounters a stranger with whom he quarrels. The quarrel turns to violence and Oedipus ends up killing the stranger, who is, of course, his real father.

The first part of the prophecy has come true. Ignorant of what he has done, however, Oedipus continues on his way to Thebes. At the time, Thebes is under siege by a monster called the Sphinx who will not let anyone pass without them answering a riddle. Oedipus answers the riddle correctly, and the Sphinx, somewhat dramatically, kills herself. Oedipus is then rewarded for freeing the city by being given the hand of the widowed queen and becoming the new king. He has fulfilled the second part of the prophecy.

Still ignorant of what he has done, he lives happily with his new wife/mother and they have four children together. It is only after Thebes falls into ruin, plagued by the curse of Oedipus's actions, that it begins to become evident to him what he has done. His wife/mother, Jocasta, on learning of what they have done, kills herself. Oedipus doesn't kill himself, but instead blinds himself and leaves Thebes.

Importantly, in Sophocles's version of the story, the action all happens, as it were, in flashback. The play begins with Oedipus already the king of Thebes, already married to Jocasta and already having killed his father. That is to say, the actions that precipitate the situation the characters are in is told retrospectively. This should remind us of Lacan's point about the movement from being to meaning.

Freud argues that the Oedipus myth has stayed around for so long and has resonated so forcefully with generations because it echoes something we all, on some level, know from first-hand experience. It tells us something about ourselves. Each of us, Freud argues, finds ourselves at a young age in a similar situation to that of Oedipus. We are bound in a powerful amorous and affectionate relationship with our mothers, and we perceive our fathers as a rival for her affections and wish him gone. Freud's theory then narrates how this predicament is resolved. If we were to stay deadlocked in this situation or if we were to win and retain our mothers and dispense with our fathers, then we would never grow up and move on to be able to live the life of an independent adult. It is only by overcoming our desire to 'kill' our father and submitting to his intervention, his prohibiting of unbridled access to our mothers, that we can achieve the necessary separation to live our own lives.

What I am referring to here as 'moving on' necessitates what Freud calls a change in object choice. The mother has, until this point, been the primary object choice. She is everything. With the intervention of the father, we are brought to a secondary object choice. It is here that identification appears to figure. The boy, according to Freud, as he cannot defeat the father, identifies with him instead. He then adopts as his secondary object choice a stand-in (or, more realistically, a series of stand-ins) for the mother. These will be other people who resemble the mother. On the most basic level, this could mean other women. It might also mean, more specifically, other women who look like, act like or share traits or pastimes with the mother.

This all seems fairly straightforward for boys, but how does a girl get from having her mother as an object choice to having men as her object choice? Clearly, not every girl does, just as not every boy chooses women. Freud's theory at this point is decidedly heteronormative. That contentious point notwithstanding, Freud concocts an explanation which is clearly intended to resolve this theoretical stumbling point. He argues that the girl identifies with the mother but is simultaneously angry with the mother for having made her incomplete. Like the mother she lacks a penis. In her anger with the mother, she turns to the father and takes him as a secondary object choice. As this is forbidden, she then has to turn to a third object choice in the form of other people who resemble the father, i.e., other men.

As preposterous as Freud's theory might seem, we can perhaps discern some kernel of truth in it. That some parts of the theory may seem a stretch and some parts may sit badly with 21st-century perspectives isn't necessarily a reason to reject the whole thing out of hand. The idea of the Oedipus complex is used for repeated comic effect in the HBO series *Succession*, with a particularly grotesque example presented when the character of Kendall stages a 40th birthday party for himself that entails all the guests entering the party through a giant representation of his mother's vagina, while he plots his father's downfall. As Freud would be the first to point out, the comic dimension only serves to underscore the continuing relevance and continuing unacceptability of the myth.

We know that babies are very attached to their mothers, and we know that something must happen to allow that attachment to abate. The commonplace idea that children just naturally move on might seem less extreme, but it doesn't really seem terribly convincing or explanatory. At the same time, not everyone has a mother or a father. People are brought up by two dads or single mums, for example. Doesn't Freud's theory rather suppose that everyone is born into a very conventional nuclear family? Moreover, the reliance on identity as the mechanism predicting one's choice of type of sexual partner or love interest appears to, if not foreclose the possibility of same-sex partners, at the very least abnormalise this as a choice.

Lacan, heeding these points, reconfigures the theory, focusing more on the structures than adherence to the content of the myth. In part, what Lacan is doing here, as he does so often, is turning us away from the temptation of imaginary identification, of getting caught up in a narrative, and focusing us instead on an impersonal structure. Where Freud's theory appears to suppose a triad of mother, baby and father, Lacan instead suggests that there is mother (who need not be the biological mother), baby and something else. This something else might be the father, it might be another man, it might be another woman or it might the mother's job or the TV or her gym routine. What Lacan is drawing our attention to is that the significant point for the child is that the mother desires something else, something other than the child. This intervention of the third has a number of effects. If the mother wants something other than the child or is perceived as wanting something other than the child, this would mean that the child is not it for the mother.

This also functions as a block to access to the mother. Whatever this other thing is, it is effectively getting in the way and saying, no, you can't have her, or at least can't have an exclusive right or access to her. This situation is actually, argues Lacan, essential for the child because, without it, the child would suffocate.

But nothing is straightforward and black and white. That the child is not the satisfaction of the mother's desire may mean that the child can attain that necessary space from the mother, the space that would allow it to move on and live its life, but it also means that the child is not it, that it is lacking and, as the child still desires the mother, and experiences a prohibition of this desire, there is a deprivation at work.

The child thus experiences itself as lacking both in the sense that it is not complete (without the mother) and lacking in the sense that it is not sufficient (for the mother) and it perceives that this situation arises through the intervention of another.

The productive dimension of this process aside, it will leave its mark. How exactly it leaves its mark can vary. Like Freud, Lacan argues that this process is such that it will be repressed. Like Oedipus, we choose to blind ourselves to what has transpired, to unknow what we have been part of.

Lacan focuses on the presumed intervention, what he terms the no of the father. In French, this sounds very similar to 'the name of the father' – *le non du père* and *le nom du père*. Lacan is playing on this homophony and uses the two versions interchangeably. In so doing, he is drawing our attention to the fact that there is an intervention, a prohibition, but also that this prohibition marks the advent of language, in the sense that one term (the father) comes to stand in or substitute for another (the mother's desire).

Lacan is bringing together two fundamental aspects of the symbolic order – rules and exchange – and it is this, he argues, that is the really crucial aspect of this process. The child is brought into the symbolic order and thus brought into the system or structures which will condition and constrain, but also allow, its own position.

Where in Freud's version much is made of the penis, the fact that some have one and some don't, Lacan moves away from this biologism. He retains, however, the basic structural logic he discerns in Freud. It may be too reductive to attempt to explain sexual identity and sexual object choice on the existence or non-existence of a penis but there is, Lacan is saying, something which creates the sense of a difference. He argues that this something is the lackingness that Freud's theory points too, even if it didn't quite know that it was pointing to this. The child wishes to be it for the mother, but the mother's desire is directed elsewhere. This is understood by the child as a prohibition. This prohibition divests the child of the imagined something it would have had that would have allowed it to be the satisfaction of the mother's desire. Following Freud, Lacan terms this imagined something the Phallus. He is keen to stress that by phallus he doesn't mean penis, but Lacan is presumably savvy enough to know that the term will resonate that way, regardless of what he stresses.

If this elusive something that the child discovers it does not have is the phallus, and the discovery of its lacking it is attributed to the father figure's prohibiting interjection, then it follows that this moment constitutes something like a symbolic castration, and this is how Lacan refers to it. Just as the phallus isn't the physical penis, this use of the term castration should not be understood to mean an actual physical castration, even in the sense of an anxiety about losing your actual penis. The castration Lacan talks of here is much more concerned with the production of lack, which is instituted through the fact of the mother's desire being directed elsewhere.

As we have seen earlier, the possibility of being a subject, being a speaking being, relies on our emergence in language. This emergence in language creates a kind of nostalgia for an impossible time before we emerged in language. To put this in a rather tautological way, this time before is impossible in the sense that the subject (who is always the subject of language) simply wouldn't have existed (as a subject of language) before its emergence in language. Or phrased otherwise, as we only know things in language, we couldn't know a time before language. Recall too that with language comes a structuring of experience and, in this sense, entering language is tantamount to entering into society. This is why Lacan uses the term symbolic to bring together the ideas of law, culture, tradition, morality and language.

Freud himself had grappled with this idea of the movement from a kind of animal being to a human society or culture. Much taken by the idea of myth, Freud invents his own myth to explain this movement. I stress the fact that it is a myth, and a myth invented by Freud, to underscore the fact that Freud is not claiming that this actually happened. Again, the idea of a before of language or culture could only be formulated as an idea after the advent of language and culture. It can only, then, be posited as a myth.

Freud's myth concerns what he terms a primal horde, a loose collective of proto-humans, similar in many ways to a band of gorillas. Like gorillas, there is an alpha male who jealously and aggressively maintains sole access to the females of the group. Freud refers to this figure as the primal father. The myth tells how the other, younger, less powerful males of the group band together to overthrow the primal father in order to gain access to the females. Having killed the primal father, the males, however, start to experience remorse, and instead of enjoying the access to females they had fought for, they stage a ceremony which entails eating the dead father and instituting as a rule the very prohibition that the father had enforced when alive. That is to say, they create a law banning themselves from having sex with the females of the group.

Through this myth, Freud links together a number of the ideas we have been exploring. The myth describes the advent of culture, or the move from being to meaning. Importantly, however, it posits a prohibition of incest (in-group sex) as the marker of this move to culture or society, as the first step in the invention of law. This reflects the Oedipal story, which has been so central to Freud. There too, incest is the crucial point around which what follows turns. In the Oedipal theory, it is the father's intervention that prohibits the child from having access to the mother. In the myth of the primal horde, it is the father's posthumous intervention which prohibits the brothers from gaining access to the females of the group.

As he had done with the Oedipus Complex, Lacan takes Freud's myth of the primal horde and strips it of its imaginary content,

$\exists x \overline{\varnothing x}$	$\overline{\exists x}\,\overline{\varnothing x}$
$\forall x \varnothing x$	$\overline{\forall x}\varnothing x$

reducing it, quite literally in this case, to a series of formulae. These look utterly baffling on first encounter, but they are actually quite straightforward.

Lacan (1998, p. 78)

The letters and symbols refer to a mix of standard logical notations and Lacan's own abbreviation of the phallus. $\exists$ means 'there exists,' $\forall$ means 'all,' $\varnothing$ refers to what Lacan calls the phallic function or castration (in the sense of castration that we outlined above) and x is simply a placeholder, as you use it in standard algebra. When there is a line over the top of a term, it means that this term is negated. We can then read the two pairs of statements fairly easily.

On the left-hand side, the first statement says there exists one who is not castrated. The statement under this says all *x* are castrated. This might initially sound like a contradiction. If all are castrated, then there cannot exist one who is not. The one who is not, however, is, we might say, the exception that proves the rule. If we recall Freud's myth, it makes much more sense. The primal father was not subject to the prohibition which was instituted in commemoration of his death. The prohibition is a symbolic castration of the males of the group. The primal father is not castrated. The brothers are. But, importantly, the brothers' castration is causally linked to the fact that the father is not castrated. Or, flipped the other way, the non-castration of the father is the logical predicate of the castration of the brothers. The privation of the brothers is only possible as privation on the basis of the existence of one who is not deprived.

On the other side, the top line reads there does not exist one who is not castrated. While this clearly contradicts the point above, this is not a problem. This side of the formula is describing a different group, i.e., the women. In this sense it is fairly straightforward. Where there is one male, the father, who was not castrated, all the women are castrated, in the sense that they are all, without exception, subject to the prohibition. There is no female equivalent of the primal father.

The final statement is the one that confuses and really brings something novel to the theory. Here, Lacan says that not all *x* are subject to castration. Now, we have just read that, on the female side, there is no exception, as there was on the male side. There is no female equivalent of the primal father. This being the case, then how can it also be true that not all are castrated? The secret here is in how we read the 'not all.' Not all could mean not all members of the group, but it could also mean not every part of each member. That is to say, while there is no female equivalent of the primal father, no uncastrated member of this group, no female is entirely castrated.

What would it mean to say that someone was not entirely castrated? Surely castration is, in this regard, a little like pregnancy. You can't be a bit castrated. You are either castrated or you are not. We need to keep in mind here that by castration, Lacan is referring to the institution of a lack that is produced through our emergence into the symbolic order. When he says that all the males are castrated, he is saying men are totally under the rule of the symbolic. When he says that women are not entirely castrated, he is saying that there is an aspect of the feminine position which escapes the rule of the symbolic order.

This, for Lacan, is the basis of sexual difference. It is a curious theory in that it appears to bracket off any direct dependence on genitalia or gonads, the very terms we would usually refer to as markers of sexual difference. Although Lacan was formulating this theory in the early 1970s, it is a theory that is perhaps only beginning to find its moment now, in the mid-21st century.

One of the interesting and potentially productive aspects of Lacan's theory here is that he effectively describes the two sexual positions, male and female, in such a way that they are not simply defined in opposition to each other. Conventionally, the idea of a sexual binary suggests that one side is what it is because it is not the other. This then is often drawn into an idea of complementarity, which works as an excuse to maintain the binary and all that flows from it. Men are active; women are passive. Men are hunter gatherers; women are nurturers. Men are leaders; women are more collective. Yin and yang. In each instance, the terms of the binary support each other through opposition and then work together to maintain a certain perspective on sexual difference. In Lacan's theory, however, the two terms are not defined in opposition to each other. They are each defined separately in relation to a third term, the phallus.

This leads Lacan to argue that there is in fact no relation between the sexes. Playing with words, as he is prone to do, Lacan formulates this idea in such a way that it condenses a number of related ideas. It is helpful then to work from the original French phrase he deploys, as the various meanings get a little lost in translation. Lacan declares that *il n'y a pas de rapport sexuel*. The French term *rapport* can variously mean 'rapport,' 'relation' or 'ratio.' The term *sexuel*, in this context, can then indicate both the idea of sexed positions (i.e., male or female) or sex as in the act of sex. Keeping these variations in mind, Lacan's phrase can be understood to mean that there is no relationship between the sexes but also that there is no rapport between the sexes. There is no relation between the sexes because, as we have seen, they are each determined in relation to a third term, not in relation to each other. This, and the consequent fact of this constituting a different position with regard to the symbolic order, suggests that there is no rapport between them either. This implies both an undermining of the myth of sexual complementarity and indicates an incompatible difference in our relations to language. If language is the symbolic order and men are totally under the rule of the symbolic but women are not, then there is a necessary and fundamental misalignment in terms of each position's relation to language. A crucial ramification of this point is that there is no position from which to articulate the idea of sexual difference which is not already biased. There is no neutral or outside position.

The idea that there is no sexual relation also, rather obviously, and oddly, seems to suggest that people don't have sex. Clearly, this is not the case and Lacan was the first to acknowledge that they do. He wants to argue, however, that, as there is no rapport between the sexes, when people have sex, they are somehow misaligned.

We have seen previously that *objet petit a* relates to the idea of a mythical unity which would have predated our emergence in and division by language, and we have also seen the related idea that we did seemingly enjoy such a unity in union with our mother, either *in utero* or while breastfeeding. Both of these ideas are instances of what Lacan would call fantasy.

Remember, the fundamental experience of the mirror stage is one which produces both division and a sense of incompleteness and that this, in experience, is supported and confirmed by our emergence as divided in and by language, producing the unconscious effect of longing for a lost unity or wholeness. Fantasy for Lacan is always the fantasy that this lack can be shored up, that we will find something that will make us whole, that it will all be ok in the end. This is why Lacan writes the formula of fantasy as the subject in relation to *objet petit a* ($\$\lozenge a$). The *objet petit a*, whatever its stand-in, is always posited as that which would make us complete.

One obvious instance wherein we feel this ought to be the case is in sexual or romantic relationships. Our cultures echo this idea very clearly.

As long ago as Plato, the idea was there in the myth of the origins of love as told by Aristophanes in *The Symposium*. The myth tells of how originally the Earth was peopled by creatures with four arms and legs, two faces and two sets of genitals. Curiously, in the myth the original creatures are of three types, those with what we would now understand as two sets of male genitals, those with two sets of female genitals and those with one of each. These creatures were completely happy and self-sufficient, but they threatened and angered Zeus, the king of the Gods, who struck them with lightning, severing each one in two. Humans have roamed the Earth ever since, so the myth suggests, searching for their other half, that which will make them complete again.

The attainment of *a* is, however, as we have seen, an impossibility. Whatever substitute we find to fill our lack, in one way or another, it never quite does. The children's writer Shel Silverstein captures this notion quite beautifully in his book *The Missing Piece*. The story concerns a circle with a segment missing, like a pizza with a piece cut out of it. It wanders around looking for the piece that will fit into this gap and complete it. As it does, it enjoys the world, enjoys rolling down hills, encountering a butterfly, stopping to talk to a worm, smelling a flower, but its goal is always to find its missing piece. It finds a piece that looks just right but the piece doesn't want to be its piece. It finds a piece that is a bit too small and a piece that is a bit too big. It finds a piece that fits, but it loses it. It finds a piece that fits, but it breaks it. Eventually, it finds a piece that fits just right and it is finally complete. Only, with its gap filled, it rolls too fast and can no longer enjoy the things it enjoyed before. It is complete in one sense, but its life remains incomplete in others.

The point, as if Silverstein was a Lacanian, is that incompleteness is an unavoidable structural fact. We may aspire to completeness, but complete completeness is not possible. This should echo with the point we discussed in relation to mother-child unity. While perhaps perceived as desirable, this unity is not necessarily very pleasant and we are, fundamentally, like all other animals, pleasure-seeking creatures.

This is not a novel idea. Even those most unpsychoanalytic thinkers, the Utilitarians, would agree that we spend our lives trying to maximise pleasure and minimise displeasure. The big difference between us and other animals is that we have language and hence the ability to think, plan, communicate and cooperate. This doesn't stop us seeking pleasure and seeking to minimise displeasure. It just makes it a bit more complicated. We are able to defer pleasure. We are able to judge other people's, and our own, pleasure-seeking activities. We are able to make up rules about what pleasures are acceptable pleasures and what pleasures are unacceptable pleasures.

In a kind of secondary loop, we even find pleasure in regulating or blocking other people's pleasure and, seemingly paradoxically, we even find pleasure in regulating, deferring or blocking our own pleasure or in punishing ourselves. We are able to make up entirely new pleasures or at least convince ourselves and others that we have. We create objects and pastimes that are presented as pleasurable and then these objects or pastimes become desirable simply because we have – or someone, the big Other, has – decided they should be. In the process, we could say, the actual attainment of pleasure kind of slips away.

The term Lacan tends to use for pleasure is *jouissance. Jouissance* basically translates as pleasure and is most often used in French to refer to sexual pleasure. It does, however, carry a second meaning, which is to refer to the rights one has to use, or enjoy, property. Lacan employs the term *jouissance* throughout his work (from the 1950s on), but the manner in which he uses it varies quite considerably. The sense of *jouissance* which is probably most commonly invoked emerges in the 1960s. Here, *jouissance* would be the sense of pleasure which would be (impossibly) achieved were *objet petit a* to be attained. This impossibility works on two levels. In part, the logic here is concerned with the fact that we live in language. Pure being, access to a world without language, is impossible. Yet the idea that it could or might have been possible gives rise to the idea that there is a pleasure available somewhere, somehow, that is not tainted by language. A pure pleasure in a pure being. Such a pure pleasure would be *jouissance.* A little like the ending of *The Missing Piece*, although perhaps in a slightly more dramatic form, this pure pleasure would also be destructive.

We might think of the beginning of Clive Barker's *Hellraiser.* A man buys a mysterious puzzle box which is said to have the power of unlocking access to indescribable pleasure. When he solves the puzzle, hooked chains appear, the hooks sinking into his flesh and then tearing him apart. The indescribable pleasure is not only indescribable but so intense that it is indistinguishable from pain. It is not only unbearable in the sense that it cannot be sustained or tolerated; it is unbearable in the sense that it obliterates.

This indiscernible status of *jouissance* allows us to appreciate the fact that, as Freud put it, there is something beyond the pleasure principle. We don't simply desire pleasure but are driven towards something which exceeds this.

In one sense, this can still be understood in terms of the mythical or primal unity of which we have spoken. One way we might understand this unity or this return to what is assumed to have been before would be in terms of our own disappearance or unbecoming.

This is captured in Freud's concept of death drive, which entails both a sense of returning to stasis or nothingness and a sense of destructiveness or aggression. This urge is, then, rather different from the urge we have called desire.

The term death drive is a translation of the German term *Todestrieb*. *Trieb*, in Freud's work, has tended to be translated into English as instinct. The term instinct, in English, has a strong biological connotation and would usually be understood as referring to a kind of inbuilt or hardwired response system that animals exhibit when presented with certain stimuli. The most obvious examples of instinct are perhaps flight or fight. When an animal is faced with a threat, it recourses to one of two responses: it fights or it runs away. Its instinct here is concerned with self-preservation, and the responses are hardwired in such a way that there is no deliberation. In this sense, an instinct is a short-circuit around thought. This is why we would usually consider animals more instinctual than humans. They don't think. We, on the other hand, like Descartes, think of ourselves as largely thinking things.

Lacan translates *Trieb* as *pulsion* and, in English translations of and commentaries on Lacan's work, this is usually translated as drive. *Pulsion* and drive have the advantage of not being tethered to an idea of the biological or the natural.

While Freud had touched on the notion of *Trieb*, he had, by his own account, not fully accounted for how these drives or instincts figure in psychoanalysis. Lacan then, we could say, continues this unfinished work.

Where Freud had noted various different instincts – such as a sexual instinct and the instinct for self-preservation – Lacan argues that all drives are death drives.

This can be understood in the sense that the very thing which would render us complete would also render us void, the very thing which would deliver us untold pleasure would also destroy us.

Where the idea of desire is an always fantasmatic movement towards an impossible object, sustained by surrogates which are never it, Lacan's later idea of drive concerns a circling of the black hole of *objet petit a*. Drive is sustained in this way by the lack, without ever touching on or attaining the lack. In this sense, drive can be understood as concerned with repetition. While the drive circles the *objet petit a*, it is not so much concerned with the object (which is in fact a lack), but with the movement of repetition. It is not what is circulated that counts, but what is repeated in this circulation. It is in this sense that all drives are the death drives: a movement towards nothingness.

CHAPTER SUMMARY

This chapter sought to outline Lacan's idea of sexual difference and the relationship between the sexes. The key ideas covered were:

- Freud used the story of Oedipus to explain the idea of how children develop sexed identities and succeed in transferring their affection from their mothers onto other 'object choices.'
- Lacan develops Freud's ideas but in such a way as to describe them as a logical operation rather than a story.
- Freud developed his own myth about a primal band of proto-humans to explain the idea of the prohibition of incest and the emergence of society and laws.
- Lacan again develops Freud's ideas, but again as a logical formulation rather than a story.
- Lacan's resulting formulation presents an idea of sexual difference that does not depend on the opposition male/female.
- Lacan further argues that the two sexes do not actually relate to each other.
- One conclusion we might draw from this is that the idea that a sexual partner would complete us is illusory.
- Lacan develops Freud's idea of *Trieb*/drive, arguing that all drive is ultimately death drive, a notion that combines the idea of completion with extinction which is held in abeyance by repetition.

9

SO WHAT?

If Lacan leaves us with a sense of the inevitability of lack, of our constitutive incompleteness, if he leaves us striving after an impossible object of desire, an object which is never actually it at all, or, at best, perpetually circling an absence in a perhaps soothing repetition, then we might rightly ask, what, ultimately, is the point?

Framed in terms of psychoanalytic practice, we might say that grasping this is precisely the point. Where other forms of therapy might seek to mend you, this is not the aim of psychoanalysis, at least in its Lacanian form. The very idea that we could be mended, as is hopefully obvious by now, is itself a fantasy. There would be something rather unethical, then, in an analyst working to convince you that you had or could impossibly shore up the lack. You might want (at least consciously) to have your lack shored up and, if this is the case, then it may simply be that Lacanian analysis is just not for you. No one says it has to be for everyone. Lacan was not a moralist, trying to persuade the world that it was everyone's duty to follow his way. The choice to enter analysis is always that, a choice. If we do make that choice though, then what is it we are aiming to accomplish? Or, put in a slightly different way, what would be the ends of analysis? Does it have an end? It may be unethical to collude with someone in the fantasmatic sealing of their lack, helping them to convince themselves that they are what they are not, encouraging an identification with an idea of mental health which is never truly possible, but it is surely just as unethical to trap someone in an expensive, endless circulation.

DOI: 10.4324/9781315622002-9

Lacan formulates the ends of analysis in a few different but intrinsically conjoined ways, aspects of which may now seem quite logical having read what precedes.

One way in which he talks about the ends of analysis is in what he calls traversing the fundamental fantasy. Recall that, for Lacan, whatever the specific content of our individual fantasy, it is always the fantasy of completion. Fantasy is always the subject in relation to or with *objet petit a* ($\$\lozenge a$). To traverse the fantasy is to overcome this idea that *objet petit a* could be attained. This would entail accepting, to some degree, that lack is simply what there is. This might seem a rather bleak outlook. It would seem to suggest that we need to accept that, as subjects, we need to relinquish the idea of that very thing which sustains our desire, that very thing which keeps us going. This thing may be illusory but surely keeping going is not, and if it requires an illusion to keep us going, then maybe that's not such a bad thing.

The error here is that we are focusing on only one side of the formula of fantasy, the *objet petit a*. We need to focus on the other side too.

Hopefully what you will have grasped from reading this book is that, for Lacan, it is not simply that the *objet a* is illusory or impossible (and also necessary). If we return to our discussion of the mirror stage, we should recall that a fundamental point being made is that the idea we build of our self, the idea of *I*, is necessarily mistaken. This, as we have seen, is not a case of us taking an erroneous identity and having to work through analysis to find the correct or true identity. The point Lacan is making is that there is nothing behind the 'erroneous' version. Even talking of an erroneous version in the singular is rather misleading. None of us is really singular. We are complex – in the proper sense of being made up of many parts – we are conflicting, we are contradictory and we are incomplete.

The aim of analysis, therefore, entails unshackling ourselves from these ideas we have of ourselves, which is to say, it entails overcoming all those identifications which we take to be who we are, all those identifications to which we cling, even when they prove less than beneficial.

Lacan calls this idea subjective destitution. If coming to accept that nothing will ever be it sounded bleak, then surely the idea of embracing destitution sounds even bleaker.

It helps, perhaps, to appreciate that while the French term *destitution* connotes the same sense of bleakness as the English, it also carries a sense of dismissal and departure. Moreover, we ought to hear in the term an echo of a term we have used earlier, constitution. Destitution and constitution both share the same root, the Latin *statuere*, meaning to set up, erect or make firm. *Statuere* is also the root of the word statue. The activity of destitution might then, in this context, be understood as the reversal of constitution, unestablishing what has been established, dismantling what has been set up or toppling the statue we have taken to be our self.

The third instalment of MCU's *Spider-Man* series, *Spider-Man: No Way Home*, offers an illustrative example of this. At the end of the previous instalment of the series, the news anchor, J Jonah Jameson, broadcasts faked footage of Spider-Man, framing him for the drone attack on London, before revealing his true identity as Peter Parker to the world. This revelation effects not only Peter but also his friends MJ and Ned, and all three find themselves being rejected from their places at university. Looking to undo this damage to his friends' futures, Peter asks Dr Strange to cast a spell which will make everyone forget the revelation. The spell, however, will also make MJ and Ned forget and Peter starts to confuse matters by asking Dr Strange to modify the spell. Eventually, Dr Strange stops but not before he has unwittingly opened a portal between different universes, allowing people from various different Spider-Man movies into the world of the current film.

The point here is that, in an endeavour to regain his secret, which is an essential part of his identity, Peter risked losing his relationships, which are also an essential part of his identity.

Amongst the characters brought into his world by Dr Strange's aborted spell are two previous iterations of Spider-Man/Peter Parker, played by the two actors who had played him in previous films. What we end up with then is three different instances of one character, but played overtly as three different characters. This splitting of Spider-Man can be understood as a kind of splitting of the subject. None of the three is in any sense the true Spider-Man. There is no original from which the others are derivations or deviations. Like the Lacanian subject, there is no true identity behind the assumed identities.

At the end of the film, after having dealt with the various visitors from other universes, the two interloping Peters return to their own universes and the remaining Peter and Dr Strange resolve to complete the spell they had started, to heal the rift in the multiverse and to continue to erase any memory of Peter from the world(s). Once the spell is done, Peter drops in at the coffee shop where MJ is working and Ned is enjoying a coffee. Not only do they not recognise him, as they no longer have any knowledge of him, but their lives don't actually appear to be affected by his non-existence. They both seem quite happy. MJ is still largely a loner, and Ned is still a nerd. The point is that the significance that we assume we must have in the world around us is largely imaginary.

It is largely imaginary but also symbolic. A curious element of the film that is never really picked up is that, in order to fully erase any knowledge of Peter Parker from everyone's minds, Strange would have to have removed all records of Peter too. That is to say, Peter is not simply removed from the imaginary, but must also be removed from the symbolic. The net effect of this is that, ultimately, as a true Lacanian subject, in the universe of the final scenes of the film, the universe as it is after Dr Strange's intervention, there is no Peter Parker. The character still exists, but there is no inscription of him in the world.

Of course, subjective destitution doesn't actually entail some kind of wizardly mass hypnosis. It is not concerned with the erasure of other people's memories. Rather, subjective destitution is concerned with the realignment of one's relationship with oneself, the acceptance that one's imaginary identifications are not the real of who we are, that the symbolic inscriptions that mark each of us, birth certificates, marriage certificates, passports, qualifications and social media profiles, are not who we are. But we are also not something else beyond these things. Any renunciation of identity positions will necessitate new identity positions. New positions which will also not be it.

The end of analysis is not then the assumption of a position without identity, which would in fact then just be another identity. It is the assumption of a position of subjectivity which entails the recognition that all the positions of identity you might find attaching to yourself are never you.

CHAPTER SUMMARY

This chapter sought to draw out some of the ramifications of Lacan's theory and articulate what we might understand as the point of psychoanalysis. The main ideas covered were:

- The end of psychoanalysis is not to be cured or made whole.
- The end of psychoanalysis is actually to overcome the fantasy that we might or could ever be made whole.
- This entails undoing the idea that we have constructed of ourselves.

10

SO WHAT NOW?

We have toured through some complex theory, and I have attempted to present an idea of what it is that Jacques Lacan gives us, an idea of his ideas. As noted at the very outset, Lacan's writing and teaching, and the ideas that he is conveying through his writing and teaching, are notoriously difficult. A core idea through all that you have read in the previous chapters has been the idea of the impossibility of closure, the idea of incompleteness as a necessary structural condition of our existence as speaking beings. There is an impossibility and an incompleteness too to what I have tried to capture here. I hope, however, that it has presented just enough of an idea of Lacan's teachings to allow you a way in. Should this have piqued your interest, there is a wealth of writing on Lacan that you might want to move on to.

INTRODUCTION

This book is very much intended as an entry-level text on Lacan. There are a number of other introductions to his work which cover some of the same ground but assume a bit more of a background. If this book has made you curious and you want to move to the next level, without moving too fast, particularly in terms of getting more to grips with some of the perplexing terminology Lacan and his followers use, then the following are valuable stopping points.

Homer, S. (2005) *Jacques Lacan*. London. Routledge.
Leader, D. & Groves, J. (1995) *Lacan for Beginners*. London. Icon Books.

DOI: 10.4324/9781315622002-10

If you would like to try to understand the development of Lacan's thought in the context of his own life, an invaluable read is Elizabeth Roudinesco's biography.

Roudinesco, E. (1999) *Jacques Lacan: An Outline of a Life and a History of a System of Thought*. Trans. Barbara Bray. Cambridge. Columbia University Press.

LACAN HIMSELF

Of course, at some point, if you are interested in Lacan, you should read Lacan himself. I would actually advocate moving to Lacan sooner rather than later. Reading his work can be challenging but if you take it slowly and focus on the clearings in the woods, the parts that do start to make some sense to you, you will get to grips with it. It is perhaps worth keeping in mind that, just as this book has repeatedly emphasised the impossibility of closure, there is no closure with Lacan, either in his teachings or his writings. This is also then to say that there is no singular interpretation of Lacan. I have given a version here and other texts you read will give other versions and as you read Lacan yourself you will form your own. There is also, however, a growing body of work providing guides to reading Lacan. These guides are not, and are not meant to be, definitive. They can, however, be very helpful. Chief among such guides is the four volume collection *Reading Lacan's Écrits*. Together, the four volumes provide a single, paragraph-by-paragraph commentary on each of the essays in *Écrits*, Lacan's main collection of essays.

Neill, C., Hook, D. & Vanheule, S. (eds.) (2023) *Reading Lacan's Écrits: From 'Overture' to 'Presentation on Psychical Causality'*. London. Routledge.
Hook, D., Vanheule, S. & Neill, C. (eds.) (2022) *Reading Lacan's Écrits: From 'Logical Time' to 'Response to Jean Hyppolite'*. London. Routledge.
Hook, D., Vanheule, S. & Neill, C. (eds.) (2019) *Reading Lacan's Écrits: From 'The Freudian Thing' to 'Remarks on Daniel Lagache'*. London. Routledge.

Vanheule, S., Hook, D. & Neill, C. (eds.) (2018) *Reading Lacan's Écrits: From 'Signification of the Phallus' to "Metaphor of the Subject'.* London. Routledge.

Lacan's major written works are collected together in two volumes of essays (he never wrote books) called *Écrits* (meaning writings) and *Autre Écrits* (meaning, you guessed it, other writings). Only the first of these has so far been translated into English. I discuss some aspects of the essay on the mirror stage in Chapter 4, although I only touch on a select few of the many points covered in the remarkably short essay. The essay, 'The Mirror Stage as Formative of the *I* Function as Revealed in Psychoanalytic Experience,' is a good place to start if you want to dive into Lacan. It is barely seven pages long, although, be warned, it is quite dense.

Lacan, J. (2006) *Écrits: The First Complete Translation in English.* Trans. Bruce Fink. London. Norton.

In some regards, Lacan's seminars, many of which have now been published in English translation (and almost all of which are available in excellent unofficial translations by Cormac Gallagher at http://www.lacaninireland.com/web/), are easier to read than his written work. As they are the edited transcriptions of his lectures, they tend to be less dense than the written work, but they can also seem less focused or structured. So, it is a bit swings and roundabouts.

Lacan, J. (1988a) *The Seminar of Jacques Lacan, Book I: Freud's Papers on Technique.* Trans. John Forrester. London. Norton.
Lacan, J. (1988b) *The Seminar of Jacques Lacan, Book II: The Ego in Freud's Theory and in the Technique of Psychoanalysis.* Trans. S Tomaselli. London. Norton.
Lacan, J. (1993) *The Seminar of Jacques Lacan, Book III: The Psychoses.* Trans. Russell Grigg. London. Routledge.
Lacan, J. (1920) *The Seminar of Jacques Lacan, Book IV: The Object Relation.* Trans. Adrian Price. London. Polity.
Lacan, J. (1917) *The Seminar of Jacques Lacan, Book V: The Formations of the Unconscious.* Trans. Russell Grigg. London. Polity.
Lacan, J. (1919) *The Seminar of Jacques Lacan, Book VI: Desire and Its Interpretation.* Trans. Bruce Fink. London. Polity.

Lacan, J. (1992) *The Seminar of Jacques Lacan, Book VII: The Ethics of Psychoanalysis*. Trans. Dennis Porter. London. Routledge.
Lacan, J. (2015) *The Seminar of Jacques Lacan, Book VIII: Transference*. Trans. Bruce Fink. London. Polity.
Lacan, J. (2014) *The Seminar of Jacques Lacan, Book X: Anxiety. Trans. Adrian Price*. London. Polity.
Lacan, J. (1977) *The Seminar of Jacques Lacan, Book XI: The Four Fundamental Concepts of Psychoanalysis*. Trans. Alan Sheridan. London. Hogarth.
Lacan, J. (2007) *The Seminar of Jacques Lacan, Book XVII: The Other Side of Psychoanalysis*. Trans. Russell Grigg. London. Norton.
Lacan, J. (2018) *The Seminar of Jacques Lacan, Book XIX: ... or Worse*. Trans. Adrian Price. London. Polity.
Lacan, J. (1998) *The Seminar of Jacques Lacan, Book XX: Encore, On Feminine Sexuality: The Limits of Love and Knowledge*. Trans. Bruce Fink. London. Norton.
Lacan, J. (2016) *The Seminar of Jacques Lacan, Book XXIII: The Sinthome*. Trans. Adrian Price. London. Polity.

Carol Owens edits an invaluable series of commentaries on the seminars which, like the commentaries on the *Écrits*, are exceedingly helpful as a support to find your way through the ideas in the text.

Owens, C. and Almqvist, N. (2019) *Studying Lacan's Seminars IV and V: From Lack to Desire*. London. Routledge.
Cox Cameron, O. with Owens, C. (2021) *Studying Lacan's Seminar VI: Dream, Symptom, and the Collapse of Subjectivity*. London. Routledge.

FREUD

Arguably, to really get to grips with Lacan, you also need to get to grips with Freud. Lacan, from the 1950s on, described his work as a return to Freud, and many of his essays and seminars focus on selected Freudian texts. For a fairly quick overview of Freud, you could do worse than pick up Jonathan Lear's introduction or if, again, you prefer a more biographical approach, Elizabeth Roudinesco has also written an excellent biography of Freud.

Lear, J. (2005) *Freud*. London. Routledge.
Roudineso, E. (2016) *Freud: His Time and Ours*. Trans. Catherine Porter. Cambridge. Harvard University Press.

Freud's own writings are published in a complete 24 volume set by Vintage Books. If you are looking for a place to start with Freud himself, I would recommend starting with one of the famous case studies. These give a fascinating insight into Freud's method and style of analysis.

Freud, S. (2001). Standard Edition Vol. VII. *A Case of Hysteria, Three Essays on Sexuality and Other Works.* Trans. James Strachey. London. Vintage.
Freud, S. (2001). Standard Edition Vol. X. *Two Case Histories: 'Little Hans' and the 'Rat Man'*. Trans. James Strachey. London. Vintage Books.
Freud, S. (2001). Standard Edition Vol. XVII. *An Infantile Neurosis and Other Works*. Trans. James Strachey. London. Vintage Books.

Beyond the case studies, I would steer you towards *The Interpretation of Dreams, Jokes and Their Relation to the Unconscious* and *Civilisation and Its Discontents.* The first two give more insight into some of the real nuts and bolts of how Freud understood the workings of the mind and how he developed his ideas of analysis. They are also very helpful precursors to Lacan's focus on language. *Civilisation and Its Discontents* is a good example of Freud's turn to culture and a reminder that, while psychoanalysis is primarily concerned with the psychoanalytic clinic and the individual analysand, it is always also about the wider culture in which we live. As these books were originally published in 1899, 1905 and 1930, it is worth keeping in mind that there is a wealth of theory and developments explored between the two.

Freud, S. (2001a). *Standard Edition Vol. IV. The Interpretation of Dreams. Part I.* Trans. James Strachey. London. Vintage Books.
Freud, S. (2001b). *Standard Edition Vol. V. The Interpretation of Dreams. Part II.* Trans. James Strachey. London. Vintage Books.

Freud, S. (2001c). *Standard Edition Vol. VIII. Jokes and their Relation to the Unconscious.* Trans. James Strachey. London. Vintage Books.
Freud, S. (2001d). *Standard Edition Vol. XXI. The Future of an Illusion, Civilization and Its Discontents and Other Works.* Trans. James Strachey. London. Vintage Books.

PHILOSOPHY

As will no doubt be clear from reading this book, Lacan draws not only on Freud and psychoanalysis, but he is also strongly influenced by philosophy, often engaging with philosophical texts in his seminars, as well as overtly basing some of his ideas on ideas from philosophy. We have seen this particularly in relation to Plato, Descartes and Hegel, and gaining some familiarity with these writers can be enormously beneficial in terms of understanding Lacan's own work. The key texts referred to in this book are:

Descartes, R. (1993) *Meditations on First Philosophy.* Trans. D.A. Cress. Indianapolis. Hackett.
Hegel, G.W.F. (1967) *The Phenomenology of Mind.* Trans. J.B. Baillie. New York. Harper and Row.
Plato (2008) *Symposium.* Trans. Robin Waterford. Oxford. Oxford University Press.

While Plato and Descartes are fairly straightforward, Hegel, like Lacan, can be a bit of a challenge to read. Beiser's introduction is a reasonable general introduction which gives a good oversight of the basics of Hegel's thought. One of the best books I know on Hegel is Todd McGowan's *Emancipation after Hegel: Achieving a Contradictory Revolution.* This has the advantage, in our context, of being written by a Lacanian, and it thus makes explicit some of the important connections between Hegel's and Lacan's thinking (and Freud's too).

Beiser, F. (2018) *Hegel.* London. Routledge.
MacGowan, T. (2019) *Emancipation after Hegel: Achieving a Contradictory Revolution.* Cambridge. Columbia University Press.

ETHICS

It has perhaps been evident, particularly in the closing chapter, that there is a strong ethical dimension to Lacan's thinking. This is not to say that Lacan is moralising. Quite the opposite. The ethics Lacan espouses is complex and grapples with the impossibility of any clear knowledge of what is right or wrong. Although I wrote it myself, I would still recommend my own book *Without Ground* for a clear overview of Lacan's ethical arguments. You might find a certain familiarity in the style, which you might find attractive, if you enjoyed this book. As it goes into a lot more detail than this book, it also serves as something of a stepping stone.

Neill, C. (2014) *Without Ground: Lacanian Ethics and the Assumptions of Subjectivity*. London. Palgrave.

THE CLINIC

This book only skims the surface of Lacan's ideas. As I have emphasised throughout, psychoanalysis is primarily a mode of clinical practice. If you are interested in gaining a better understanding of the theory of psychoanalysis as clinical practice, there is a wealth of books out there written by clinical practitioners which cover complex areas of the theory within the context of their clinical application. Many of these books, however, appear to be written by Lacanians for Lacanians, and they can be very difficult to read if you are not yourself a practising psychoanalyst with years of experience moving in these circles. Some of the books seem downright impenetrable. There are, however, also books written by practitioners which shine a light and do the hard work of making the ideas accessible. For a practical insight, I would recommend:

Fink, B. (1997) *A Clinical Introduction to Lacanian Psychoanalysis.* Cambridge. Harvard University Press.
Miller, M.J. (2011) *Lacanian Psychotherapy: Theory and Practical Applications*. London. Routledge.

Lacan proposes that there are three different clinical structures, effectively three different ways of being a subject. These are psychosis, neurosis and perversion. For books on psychosis, I would recommend:

Fimiani, B. (2020) *Psychosis and Extreme States: An Ethic for Treatment.* London. Palgrave.
Rogers, A.G. (2016) *Incandescent Alphabets: Psychosis and the Enigma of Language.* London. Routledge.
Vanheule, S. (2014) *The Subject of Psychosis: A Lacanian Perspective.* London. Palgrave.

For perversion:

Swales, S. (2012) *Perversion: A Lacanian Psychoanalytic Approach to the Subject.* London. Routledge.

As neurosis, both in its obsessional and its hysterical forms, is the most numerically typical structure, often the more general books on Lacanian clinical ideas are focused there. Possibly, for this reason, there seem to be less books discretely focused on these structures. This situation will hopefully change with time.

ŽIŽEK

The growth in interest in Lacan and, arguably, the subsequent growth in literature on Lacan can be traced, at least in part, to the advent of a Slovenian philosopher in the 1990s. Slavoj Žižek succeeded in popularising Lacanian ideas, bringing them, to some extent, into the mainstream. Through his application of Lacan to contemporary politics, ideology and film, he succeeded in making these ideas more accessible than they had seemed before. Žižek does, however, have two rather distinct modes of writing. He has his more accessible, often film-focused, works and he has his more challenging, more philosophical works. It is also worth noting that, while Lacan is a massive influence on Žižek, some of his works are more obviously Lacanian than others. My recommended starting point for Žižek, particularly in the context of having read this book, would be his 1989 book *The Sublime Object of Ideology*. Beyond that, the collection of essays, *Interrogating the Real* is a good access point for a range of his arguments. For the more filmic Žižek, I would recommend his books on Lynch and Kieślowski.

Žižek, S. (1989a) *The Sublime Object of Ideology*. London.Verso.
Žižek, S. (1989b) *Interrogating the Real: Selected Writings.* Edited by Rex Butler and Scott Stephens. London. Bloomsbury.
Žižek, S. (2000) *The Art of the Ridiculous Sublime: On David Lynch's Lost Highway.* Washington. Washington University Press.
Žižek, S. (2001) *The Fright of Real Tears: Krzysztof Kieślowski Between Theory and Post-Theory*. London. The British Film Institute.

Of his more philosophically focused work, the true magnum opus is perhaps 2012's *Less Than Nothing*, although I would recommend a few others too.

Žižek, S. (1993) *Tarrying with the Negative: Kant, Hegel, and the Critique of Ideology*. Duke University Press.
Žižek, S. (1996) *The Indivisible Remainder: Essays on Schelling and Related Matters.* London. Verso.
Žižek, S. (2006) *The Parallax View*. Cambridge. MIT Press.
Žižek, S. (2012) *Less Than Nothing: Hegel and the Shadow of Dialectical Materialism*. London. Verso.

It is worth noting that Žižek is a prolific writer whose engagement with the political and cultural world is always very up to date. His recent works are, therefore, in some regards, always the most relevant to read.

Žižek, S. (2022) *Surplus Enjoyment: A Guide for the Non-perplexed.* London. Bloomsbury.

FILM

From as early as the 1970s, Lacan was inspiring film theorists, with many of the great film theorists, such as Laura Mulvey, Christian Metz and Stephen Heath, having a clear stamp of Lacan's influence on their work. Lacan-inspired film theory has, however, developed significantly since those days, in part due to the more widespread availability and translation of Lacan's work and in part due to the increase in Lacan scholarship more generally and the film theory dimension of this in particular. For a good overview and application of the earlier use of Lacan in film theory, you should seek out a copy of Michael Westlake and Rob Lapsley's *Film Theory: An Introduction*. For more recent applications and developments of Lacanian Film Theory, below are some of the best.

Bristow, D. (2018) *2001: A Space Odyssey and Lacanian Psychoanalytic Theory*. London. Palgrave.
Lapsley, R. & Westlake, M. (1988) *Film Theory: An Introduction*. Manchester. Manchester University Press.
McGowan, T. (2007a) *The Impossible David Lynch*. New York. Columbia University Press.
McGowan, T. (2007b) *The Real Gaze: Film Theory after Lacan*. Albany. State University of New York Press.
Neill, C. (ed.) (2020) *Lacanian Perspectives on Blade Runner 2049*. London. Palgrave.
Tyrer, B. (2016) *Out of the Past: Lacan and Film Noir.* London. Palgrave.

RACE

One significant failing of Lacan's theory is that it does appear to be a particularly white theory. Lacan engages very little with questions of race, and, despite the nuance he introduces in terms of different modes of being for different clinical structures and different sexual positions, it is difficult not to see his work as rather flat when it comes to race. The subject of Lacanian theory does appear, unwittingly, to be the white subject. Despite, or rather, perhaps, because of, this, Lacan's ideas have started to be taken up to consider some of the complex issues of race in our culture, not least the issue of race in psychoanalytic theory itself. By far the most significant of the works in this area, and really one of the most significant books in Lacanian theory *per se*, is David Marriott's *Lacan Noir.* Beyond Marriott – and possibly advisably before you try to read Marriot – Derek Hook and Sheldon George's collection *Lacan and Race* is an excellent primer on this topic, as is George's own *Trauma and Race*.

George, S. (2016) *Trauma and Race: A Lacanian Study of African American Racial Identity*. Waco. Baylor University Press.

Hook, D. & Sheldon, G. (2021) *Lacan and Race: Racism, Identity, and Psychoanalytic Theory*. London. Routledge.
Marriott, D. (2021) *Lacan Noir: Lacan and Afro-pessimism*. London. Palgrave.

SEX AND GENDER

Unsurprisingly, given the centrality of the question of sex to psychoanalysis, there have, over the years, been many books written on gender and sex from a Lacanian perspective. These include some excellent books focusing on the feminine, such as Elizabeth Grosz's *Jacques Lacan: A Feminist Introduction*, on the masculine, such as Anthony Easthope's *What a Man's Gotta Do*, and on the (impossible) relation between the two, such as Renata Salecl's *(Per)Versions of Love and Hate.*

What is perhaps evident here, and is perhaps evident too in the book you have just read, is a tendency to still think of sex (or gender) in terms of a binary. There is something of an open discussion as to the extent to which Lacan is conforming to a binary in his work, particularly in his later work. This is not simply a case of debating what Lacan said or what he meant. It is also a question of where we can usefully go with and from Lacan's theory. When Lacan spoke of a return to Freud, one of the things he was flagging was Freud's perpetual questioning, his openness to rethink his own ideas and to clearly acknowledge the fact that he didn't have all the answers, that he hadn't produced a complete (and thus sealed) theory. In returning to Freud, Lacan was emphasising this element in his own work too. This being the case, if we are to read Lacan in a Lacanian fashion, we should always read it as open to question, as ready to be developed. One important and topical area to which this applies is the question of gender identity. The best two books in this area are by Patricia Gherovici.

Easthope, A. (2016) *What a Man's Gotta Do: The Masculine Myth in Popular Culture*. London. Routledge.
Gherovici, P. (2010) *Please Select Your Gender: From the Invention of Hysteria to the Democratizing of Transgenderism*. London. Routledge.
Gherovici, P. (2017) *Transgender Psychoanalysis: A Lacanian Perspective on Sexual Difference*. London. Routledge.

Grosz, E. (1990) *Jacques Lacan: A Feminist Introduction.* London. Routledge.
Salecl, R. (2000) *(Per)Versions of Love and Hate.* London. Verso.

CULTURE AND POLITICS

For a general consideration of Lacanian theory as a tool for engaging with politics, there is none better than Yannis Stavrakakis's *Lacan and the Political.* The other texts listed below take up specific aspects of culture and politics, and each, in their different ways, offers fascinating insights into how we can use Lacanian theory productively to think about our world and how the theory can continue to be developed. These include considerations of social media (Flisfeder), AI (Millar), literature (Rabaté), the environment (Burnham and Kingsbury) or psychoanalysis itself (Webster).

Burnham, C. & Kingsbury, P. (2021) *Lacan and the Environment.* London. Palgrave.
Matt Flisfeder, M. (2021) *Algorithmic Desire: Toward a New Structuralist Theory of Social Media.* Northwestern University Press.
Millar, I. (2021) *The Psychoanalysis of Artificial Intelligence.* London. Palgrave.
Rabaté, J.-M. (2001) *Jacques Lacan: Psychoanalysis and the Subject of Literature.* London. Routledge.
Webster, J. (2011) *The Life and Death of Psychoanalysis: On Unconscious Desire and Its Sublimation.* London. Divided Publishing.

YOUTUBE

Beyond the printed word, another valuable way to engage with Lacan's ideas is through YouTube. Among the many videos you will find there explaining or engaging with aspects of Lacan's thought, the following three channels are recommended. The first offers some engaging, stand-alone videos on key aspects of Lacan's thought. The second is a mix of short concept-based videos and interviews with Lacanian scholars. The last is a discussion channel where you can see videos of top Lacanians presenting and engaging in discussion about their current work. This latter channel is actually recordings of a monthly online seminar, which I host, and which you can attend for free on the last Thursday of every month. If reading this basic guide to Lacan has got you interested, then why not join us?

https://www.youtube.com/c/lacanonline
https://www.youtube.com/channel/UCzdZyq2SC9BtMn3fLT-knIMQ
https://www.youtube.com/c/LacanInScotland

GLOSSARY

Agalma – agalma technically refers to a statue, or specifically a statue representing a God. In his Symposium, Plato uses the term to refer to that mysterious something in someone that causes you to fall in love with them. It is this sense that Lacan develops. Agalma can be understood as one of a number of partial variants of the concept of *objet petit a*.

Alienation – alienation refers primarily to the idea of being divided from ourselves due to our existence in language.

Separation – separation refers primarily to the manner in which the child experiences itself as distinct from the mother. Importantly, for Lacan, separation does not so much imply a prior state of union as it does the fantasmatic assumption of a prior state of union. That is to say, it is the experience of separation that gives rise to the supposition of a previous state of not being separated. Separation is one of the manifestations of lack.

Borromean knot – the Borromean Knot is a topographical figure entailing three entwined rings, the cutting of any one of which will result in the separation of all three. Lacan uses the Borromean Knot to represent the fact that no one of the three realms of the symbolic, the imaginary and the real can be separated without this causing the coming apart of all three. That is to say, one's experience of the world is maintained through an interaction of the symbolic, the imaginary and the real. The three realms not being held together would be one way of describing psychosis.

Castration – castration, in Lacan's usage, refers to the perceived imposition of a lackingness, specifically the child's discovery that it does not have what it would take to completely satisfy its mother's desire. Castration is also used to describe the effect of our entry into language and the lack that this institutes. The two uses are actually bound together and, in this sense, are really one.

Conscious – the conscious is one of the three psychical elements in Freud's first topology. The other two being the pre-conscious and the unconscious. Consciousness is linked to perception and refers to the fleeting presence of thoughts as we are aware of them.

Desire – desire for Lacan is closely linked to lack, and thus to *objet petit a*. Crucially, desire, for Lacan, is always unconscious desire.

Drive – drive is the English translation of the French term *pulsion*, which, in turn, is the translation of the German term used by Freud, *Trieb*. *Trieb* is conventionally translated in English as 'instinct,' but the term as used by Freud doesn't always carry the biological connotation that instinct implies. Like desire, drive is related to *objet petit a*. Where desire aims at *objet petit a*, drive aims to circulate it. Following Freud, Lacan refers to a number of different drives, or partial drives – the anal drive, oral drive, scopic drive and the invocatory drive – but he also argues that all drives are ultimately the death drive.

Foreclosure – foreclosure is one of three modes of repression, the other two being denial and disavowal. Lacan articulates each mode of repression to a different clinical structure. Foreclosure is the mode of repression associated with psychosis. It implies that the repressed content has been entirely shut out, as though it never existed.

Imaginary – the imaginary is one of the three realms of experience, the other two being the symbolic and the real. The imaginary is the basis of identification and is closely related to the mirror stage.

Hysteria – hysteria is one of two forms of neurosis, the other being obsessional neurosis. Lacan argues that hysteria is typical of women, while obsessional neurosis is typical of men. This, however, does not mean that men cannot be hysterics. Hysteria is typified by questioning, particularly of authority.

Jouissance – jouissance is a French term meaning pleasure. It is usually used with reference to sexual pleasure but can also be used to refer to the rights one has to make use of, or enjoy, a property. Jouissance can be used to refer to an extreme pleasure, a pleasure bordering on or indistinguishable from pain, and it is often in this sense that Lacan uses it.

Mirror stage – the mirror stage refers to our formation of an identity through an encounter with an external image, most typically our own image reflected in a mirror. Lacan describes this in terms of an experience of early childhood, but the process is ultimately endless as we continue to reinforce our identity through this mirroring process throughout our lives. Crucial to the idea of the mirror stage is the fact that the image taken to be our self is always radically different from our self, even when it is our own reflection. A reflection is only a reflection, and is always to a large extent a distortion.

Name-of-the-father/no of the father – these two terms sound identical in French (*nom du père* and *non du père*). They refer to the conjoined intervention of the father figure which both prohibits access to the mother and ushers the child into language.

Neurosis – neurosis is one of three clinical categories used by Lacan, the other two being psychosis and perversion. Each clinical category is associated with a different mode of repression. The mode of repression associated with neurosis is denial. This suggests that the repressed material is pushed out of consciousness but can return.

Objet petit a – *objet petit a* is one of the key terms in Lacan's theory, referring both to the fact that we are constitutively lacking and to the fantasised thing that would make good this lack.

Obsessional neurosis – obsessional neurosis is one of two forms of neurosis, the other being hysteria or hysterical neurosis. Lacan argues that obsessional neurosis is most typical of men, while hysteria is more typical of women. The obsessional neurotic is fully within the symbolic order and, in a sense then, is not fully alive.

Phallus – where Freud had referred to the penis, Lacan prefers to use the term phallus and seeks to distinguish it in this way from the body part. The phallus, for Lacan, operates in imaginary, symbolic and real modes and refers to the absence which determines our incompleteness or castration.

Point de capiton – *points de capiton* are the buttons used by upholsterers to stop the stuffing in cushions from moving around. Lacan borrows this term to refer to the punctuating points in speech (or writing) which allow meaning to settle. Any sentence can be added to with more words which will alter the meaning of a sentence. The *point de capiton* is the point at which a stable meaning seems to have been found, although this can always be altered or inverted by further words. The classic example here is the negating addition of the word 'not' to sentences in the film *Wayne's World*.

The preconscious – Freud's first topography posits three elements of the psyche; the conscious, the preconscious and the unconscious. The preconscious refers to all those ideas or memories that we are not currently consciously thinking about but to which we have easy access.

Psychosis – psychosis is one of three clinical structures. While Lacan's use of the term psychosis necessarily shares something with the psychiatric use of the term, the fact that the two disciplines are based on radically different understandings of the mind or the subject means that the way in which the term psychosis is used is also quite different. In his later seminars, Lacan relates psychosis to the Borromean Knot, the interlocking rings of the symbolic, imaginary and real. Psychosis, Lacan argues, is the result of the rings not being locked together. Psychosis can also be understood in relation to the idea of lack, in that the psychotic forecloses their lackingness, operating as though it doesn't exist. In this sense, psychosis can be understood as characterised by certainty.

The Real – the real is one of the three realms of experience, along with the symbolic and the imaginary. The real refers to those things we don't know, things which are beyond current knowledge or for which there are no words or concepts. It also refers to the inherent gaps in language, the fact that it is never possible to say something completely or say it all.

Repression – repression refers to the fact of something having become unconscious.

Sexuation – sexuation refers to the process by which we assume sexual positions or identities.

Signifier – a signifier is the generalised form of any word or phrase (as opposed to the specific instance of its being said or written).

Signified – the signified is the idea conveyed by a signifier.

Subject – the term subject refers broadly to the idea of person. It carries the connotation, however, of being under the power of something, in the sense that in monarchies, for example, people are referred to as subjects of the crown or we are all subject to the laws of the country in which we reside.

Surplus jouissance – surplus jouissance refers to a supposed enjoyment that others have that I don't have.

Symbolic – the symbolic is one of the three realms of experience, alongside the imaginary and the real. The symbolic refers to the structuring and rule governing aspects of our experience and would include language, law, social structures, etc.

The unconscious – the unconscious is one of the three elements of the psyche in Freud's first topography, alongside the conscious and the preconscious. In the classic Freudian usage, it refers to the repository of repressed ideas. In Lacan's usage, it is more closely linked to language. In fact, Lacan argues that the unconscious is structured like a language. Used without the article, unconscious functions as an adjective to refer to those ideas which are not conscious.

BIBLIOGRAPHY

Aquinas, T. (1988) *On Politics and Ethics*. Trans. P. Sigmund. London. Norton.

Aquinas, T. (2008) *Selected Philosophical Writings*. Trans. Timothy McDermott. Oxford. Oxford University Press.

Aristotle (2008) *Physics*. Trans. David Bostock. Oxford. Oxford University Press.

Augustine (2003) *Confessions*. Trans. R.S. Pine-Coffin. London. Penguin.

Boothby, R. (2001) *Freud as Philosopher: Metapsychology after Lacan*. London. Routledge.

Coleridge, S.T. (1983) *Biographia Literaria*. Princeton: Princeton University Press.

Descartes, R. (1993) *Meditations on First Philosophy*. Trans. D.A. Cress. Indianapolis. Hackett.

Fink, B. (1995) *The Lacanian Subject: Between Language and Jouissance*. Princeton. Princeton University Press.

Freud, S. (2001) Standard Edition London. Vintage Books.

- Vol. I Pre-Psycho-Analytic Publications and Unpublished Drafts (1886–1899).
- Vol. II Studies in Hysteria (1893–1895). By Josef Breuer and S. Freud.
- Vol. III Early Psycho-Analytic Publications (1893–1899).
- Vol. IV The Interpretation of Dreams (I) (1900).
- Vol. V The Interpretation of Dreams (II) and On Dreams (1900–1901).
- Vol. VI The Psychopathology of Everyday Life (1901).
- Vol. VII A Case of Hysteria, Three Essays on Sexuality and Other Works (1901–1905).
- Vol. VIII Jokes and Their Relation to the Unconscious (1905).
- Vol. IX Jensen's 'Gradiva,' and Other Works (1906–1909).
- Vol. X The Cases of 'Little Hans' and the Rat Man' (1909).
- Vol. XI Five Lectures on Psycho-Analysis, Leonardo and Other Works (1910).
- Vol. XII The Case of Schreber, Papers on Technique and Other Works (1911–1913).

- Vol. XIII Totem and Taboo and Other Works (1913–1914).
- Vol. XIV On the History of the Psycho-Analytic Movement, Papers on Meta-Psychology and Other Works (1914–1916).
- Vol. XV Introductory Lectures on Psycho-Analysis (Parts I and II) (1915–1916).
- Vol. XVI Introductory Lectures on Psycho-Analysis (Part III) (1916–1917).
- Vol. XVII An Infantile Neurosis and Other Works (1917–1919).
- Vol. XVIII Beyond the Pleasure Principle, Group Psychology and Other Works (1920–1922).
- Vol. XIX The Ego and the Id and Other Works (1923–1925).
- Vol. XX An Autobiographical Study, Inhibitions, Symptoms and Anxiety, Lay Analysis and Other Works (1925–1926).
- Vol. XXI The Future of an Illusion, Civilization and Its Discontents and Other Works (1927–1931).
- Vol. XXII New Introductory Lectures on Psycho-Analysis and Other Works (1932–1936).
- Vol. XXIII Moses and Monotheism, An Outline of Psycho-Analysis and Other Works (1937–1939).

Hegel, G.W.F. (1967) *The Phenomenology of Mind*. Trans. J.B. Baillie. New York. Harper and Row.

Hook, D., Vanheule, S. & Neill, C. (eds.) (2019) *Reading Lacan's Écrits: From 'The Freudian Thing' to 'Remarks on Daniel Lagache'*. London. Routledge.

Hook, D., Vanheule, S. & Neill, C. (eds.) (2022) *Reading Lacan's Écrits: From 'Logical Time' to 'Response to Jean Hyppolite'*. London. Routledge.

Kafka, F. (1953) *The Trial*. Trans. Wills and Edwin Muir. London. Penguin.

Kant, I. (1965) *Critique of Pure Reason*. Trans. N. Kemp Smith. New York. St. Martin's Press.

Lacan, J. (1988a) *The Seminar of Jacques Lacan, Book I: Freud's Papers on Technique*. Trans. John Forrester. London. Norton.

Lacan, J. (1988b) *The Seminar of Jacques Lacan, Book II: The Ego in Freud's Theory and in the Technique of Psychoanalysis*. Trans. S. Tomaselli. London. Norton.

Lacan, J. (1993) *The Seminar of Jacques Lacan, Book III: The Psychoses*. Trans. Russell Grigg. London. Routledge.

Lacan, J. (1920) *The Seminar of Jacques Lacan, Book IV: The Object Relation*. Trans. Adrian Price. London. Polity.

Lacan, J. (1917) *The Seminar of Jacques Lacan, Book V: The Formations of the Unconscious*. Trans. Russell Grigg. London. Polity.

Lacan, J. (1919) *The Seminar of Jacques Lacan, Book VI: Desire and Its Interpretation*. Trans. Bruce Fink. London. Polity.

Lacan, J. (1992) *The Seminar of Jacques Lacan, Book VII: The Ethics of Psychoanalysis*. Trans. Dennis Porter. London. Routledge.

Lacan, J. (2015) *The Seminar of Jacques Lacan, Book VIII: Transference*. Trans. Bruce Fink. London. Polity.

Lacan, J. (2014) *The Seminar of Jacques Lacan, Book X: Anxiety*. Trans. Adrian Price. London. Polity.

Lacan, J. (1977) *The Seminar of Jacques Lacan, Book XI: The Four Fundamental Concepts of Psychoanalysis*. Trans. Alan Sheridan. London. Hogarth.

Lacan, J. (2007) *The Seminar of Jacques Lacan, Book XVII: The Other Side of Psychoanalysis*. Trans. Russell Grigg. London. Norton.

Lacan, J. (2018) *The Seminar of Jacques Lacan, Book XIX: … or Worse*. Trans. Adrian Price. London. Polity.

Lacan, J. (1998) *The Seminar of Jacques Lacan, Book XX: Encore, On Feminine Sexuality: The Limits of Love and Knowledge*. Trans. Bruce Fink. London. Norton.

Lacan, J. (2016) *The Seminar of Jacques Lacan, Book XXIII: The Sinthome*. Trans. Adrian Price. London. Polity.

Lacan, J. (2006) Écrits: The First Complete Translation in English. Trans. Bruce Fink. London. Norton.

Lear, J. (2005) *Freud*. London. Routledge.

Lear, E. (2014) *Edward Lear's Book of Nonsense*. London. Usborne.

Locke, J. (1975) *An Essay Concerning Human Understanding*. Oxford. Oxford University Press.

Neill, C., Hook, D. & Vanheule, S. (eds.) (2023) *Reading Lacan's Écrits: From 'Overture' to 'Presentation on Psychical Causality'*. London. Routledge.

Neill, C. (2014) Without Ground: Lacanian Ethics and the Assumptions of Subjectivity. London. Palgrave.

Nietzsche, F. (1994/1887) *On the Genealogy of Morality*. Trans. C. Diethe. Cambridge. Cambridge University Press.

Plato (2008) *Symposium*. Trans. Robin Waterford. Oxford. Oxford University Press.

Roudinesco, E. (1999) *Jacques Lacan: An Outline of a Life and a History of a System of Thought*. Trans. Barbara Bray. Cambridge. Columbia University Press.

Roudineso, E. (2016) *Freud: His Time and Ours*. Trans. Catherine Porter. Cambridge. Harvard University Press.

Salecl, R. (ed.) (2000) *Sexuation*. Durham. Duke University Press.

Schelling, F. (1978) *System of Transcendental Idealism*. Charlottesville. University of Virginia Press.

Silverstein, S. (1978) *The Missing Piece*. London. Harper Collins.

Sophocles (1984) *The Three Theban Plays: Antigone, Oedipus The King, Oedipus at Colonus*. Trans. R. Fagles. London. Penguin.

Vanheule, S., Hook, D. & Neill, C. (eds.) (2018) *Reading Lacan's Écrits: From 'Signification of the Phallus' to "Metaphor of the Subject'*. London. Routledge.

Film and TV

Hellraiser (1987) Directed by Clive Barker. Film Futures. UK.
Spider-Man: No Way Home (2021) Directed by Jon Watts. Columbia Pictures/ Marvel Studios. USA.
That Obscure Object of Desire (1977) Directed by Luis Bunuel. Greenwich Film. France/Spain.
The Matrix (1999) Directed by the Wachowskis. Warner Bros. USA.
Wayne's World (1992) Directed by Penelope Spheeris. Paramount Pictures. USA.

TV Shows

'Too Much Birthday' (2021) *Succession*, Season 3, Episode 7. HBO. USA
Euphoria (2019 – present) HBO. USA.

Song

The Who (1965) 'My Generation', *The Who Sing My Generation*. Decca. London.

INDEX